The ABC's of
Nutrition & Supplements
for Prostate Cancer

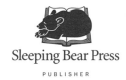

Sleeping Bear Press

PUBLISHER

The ABC's of

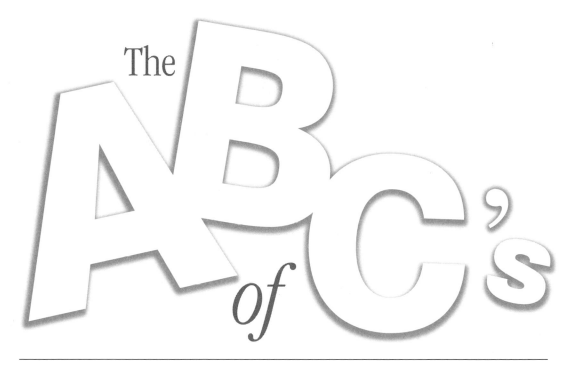

Nutrition & Supplements

for Prostate Cancer

By Mark A. Moyad, M.P.H.

Sleeping Bear Press
310 North Main Street, Suite 300
P.O. Box 20
Chelsea, Michigan 48118
www.sleepingbearpress.com

Illustrations by Patrick J. Gloria

Printed and bound in The United States.
10 9 8 7 6 5 4 3 2 1

Moyad, Mark A.
ABC's of nutrition and supplements for prostate cancer /
by Mark Moyad
p. cm.
Includes bibliographical references and index.
ISBN 1-886947-69-4
1. Prostate —Cancer—Diet therapy. 2. Dietary supplements.
I. Moyad, Mark II. Title.
RC280.P7M692000
616.99'463—dc21

99-18425
CIP

"To all of the individuals who are objectively attempting to combine conventional and alternative medicine—you are an inspiration."

—Mark Moyad, M.P.H.

"In all fighting, the direct method may be used for joining battle, but indirect methods will be needed in order to secure victory. The direct and the indirect lead on to each other in turn. It is like moving in a circle—you never come to an end. Who can exhaust the possibilities of their combination?"

—Chinese philosopher and general Sun Tzu
from *The Art of War* (500 b.c.)

Preface

It seems these days that everyone is talking about finding a cure for cancer. While it is frustrating that an answer hasn't already been discovered, we need to maintain a positive focus on locating reliable information and solutions. It can sometimes be tempting to blame others for not already having a cure; however, we'll be much better off in the long run if we resist and forge ahead. We all have an important role to play in maintaining our health, as well as providing an avenue for healthier future generations.

Let's begin by discussing the overall realities of cancer and the specifics of prostate cancer. For approximately 20 years researchers have agreed that about one-third of cancers are related to diet, one-third are related to tobacco, and the other one-third are due to unknown causes or a variety of factors. Regardless, this means that two-thirds, or 66%, of cancers are preventable. It's that simple. Just think of the tremendous time, energy, and funding we could devote to finding a cure for the remaining unknown cancer occurrences if the preventable cancers were eliminated.

Percentage of Cancer Deaths That Can Be Prevented By Dietary Change			
Type of Cancer	Doll-Peto (1981)	Willett (1994)	Overall Range of All Studies
Breast	50	50	20–80
Colon/Rectum	90	70	50–80
Endometrium	50	50	50–80
Gall Bladder	50	50	50–80
Larynx, bladder, cervix, mouth, pharynx, esophagus	20	20	10–30
Lung	20	20	10–30
Pancreas	50	50	10–50
Prostate	20	75	20–80
Stomach	35	35	30–70
Other Types	10	10	—
Total	**35**	**32**	**20–42**

Adapted from N. J. Nelson

Approximately one-third of all cancers can be prevented through diet.

In the fall of 1997 nutrition experts from around the world met to report their findings on the relationship between cancer occurrence and diet. Guess what? They too, came to the conclusion, based on medical research throughout the years, that about one-third of cancers (and maybe more) could be avoided by dietary change alone.

If more time were devoted to educating people about how to reduce cancer risk—and/or, once diagnosed, how to reduce their chances of further progression of the disease—the result would be a healthier and more productive society. This, in part, is why I have dedicated my life to the study of nutrition for cancer. Through the process of education we may be able to create a society that will never again have to experience the early loss of a loved one to cancer.

A few of my past experiences are what eventually led me to specialize in nutrition and supplements for cancer prevention and treatment. In 1976 I spent time traveling with my father in his native country, Iran. It was in Iran that I learned about people who died from diseases that could have been prevented if only someone had possessed the proper knowledge. I was dumbfounded by this discovery.

In the late '70s and early '80s I traveled to Vienna, Austria, on a regular basis to visit my mother's family. Here, for the first time, I heard about the alternative medicines that people took to remedy anything from the common cold to cancer. In addition, the lifestyle in Austria was so very different from the one I was used to at the time. Everyone gathered for meals at one table and no one seemed in a hurry to finish eating and rush off to another activity. I never saw a fast food restaurant; I spent hours talking to others without ever even considering watching the television; we all walked a lot; the whole town was closed on Sundays; we bought the local newspaper from a container with no lock—it was all so different from my life in the United States.

I attended the University of South Florida, College of Public Health from 1989-1992, where two constant themes were echoed in all my classes: prevention and education. I also assisted in the State of Florida's investigation of the L-tryptophan problem. (You may recall that L-tryptophan was a dietary supplement that caused many individuals to become seriously ill when unfortunately—and accidentally—some of the bottles became tainted with a compound that was poisonous to the body.) I also taught a health class to children at a local school in Tampa. We learned together that it was never too early and always absolutely necessary to focus on healthy behaviors.

While I was still in school I had the opportunity to visit Japan, Singapore,

Malaysia, and Thailand. That trip was probably the most valuable of my career to date. I observed some of the healthiest and least healthy people in the world. Many had horrible infectious diseases that I didn't know even existed. I was convinced that I hadn't known about them because the United States was immune from such problems. I thought Americans died mostly from chronic diseases such as heart disease or cancer, and certainly not from any of the terrible diseases I saw on my trip.

While helplessly watching a very dear member of my family die from cancer, I decided to specialize in the field of cancer research. Shortly after I began my research I realized what was confirmed by others—that a great many instances of cancer could have been prevented through diet. Please don't misunderstand me: I am not saying that everyone who has cancer could have prevented it. This is not my message at all. What I am saying is that knowledge is available today that could help prevent a large number of occurrences. The dissemination of this information remains a complex issue. It will take time, education, and research, and in the end the responsibility will lie on our shoulders (yours and mine) to learn the principles of healthy eating and incorporate them into our daily lives.

I believe this is one of the most exciting areas of medicine, one with an unlimited future. We have already begun to use this knowledge in our war against cancer, and we must not cease our efforts in this area. While we may still experience some of the same diseases I observed in my early trips abroad, at least we now have medical proof that diet can prevent some types of cancer. I am convinced that whatever you do in life can be used as a learning opportunity for the rest of your life. It all boils down to your perception and how willing you are to be open-minded. I played college basketball for two years at the College of Wooster, in Ohio. Cancer treatment should model itself after some of our athletic coaching principles. Wait—no, I'm not crazy! Let me explain. When I played basketball I was in the best physical condition of my life. In addition, the coach had us in the best mental shape of our lives. He was a tremendous motivator and convinced us that we could accomplish anything. It didn't matter if we lost miserably to our opponents, we were always ready physically and mentally to meet our nemesis.

These same principles need to be applied to the prevention and treatment of cancer. In the past, patients simply appeared for scheduled surgeries, radiation, and chemotherapy, etc., asked no questions, and waited on the sidelines for the outcome of their treatment. Although this is beginning to change, I hope to play a role in a much greater expansion of this new approach to cancer treatment. Patients need to be in the best physical and mental condition of their lives before, during, and after treatment. No one should be treated as a passive participant in a situation that effects the length and quality of his or her life. Patients need to understand that part of the responsibility for their health depends on them. They need tools in order to become active participants in their healing. These tools include dietary information, advice on supplements, meditation, and other alternative treatments. If a person is physically and mentally ready for treatment, better decisions will be made and they will have tremendous peace knowing they have done everything possible to help themselves.

Another interesting thing that taught me a valuable lesson, happened to me while in college. My first published medical article was about Gossypol, a natural product found in cottonseed oil. It was a fascinating story, Gossypol was first discovered when women in China who used a lot of cottonseed oil for cooking had trouble becoming pregnant. It became such a problem that the Chinese government investigated the situation and determined that there was a compound in the cottonseed oil that caused men to become temporarily sterile. The Gossypol pill never made it to the U.S. market because of the side effects, but I had learned a valuable lesson: Mother Nature provides us with some powerful natural elixirs—we simply have to find out where she hides them.

In 1994 the Dietary and Supplement Act was passed. I entered Wayne State University Medical School, in Detroit, Michigan in 1995. At about the same time I entered medical school the interest rose again slightly in the use of nutrition and alternative medicines for cancer prevention and treatment. This interest has continued over the last few years, and depending on whom you talk to now, almost half of all cancer patients have tried one or more types of alternative medicine. This is FANTASTIC! More individuals are playing an active role in their health care. The finest methods of both conventional and alternative medicine are being combined, thereby providing the best of both worlds for patients. This provides the best chance of surviving or of preventing cancer.

I would be remiss if I did not offer a word of caution regarding alternative medicine. There are a number of individuals who are ready, willing, and able to take advantage of the desperation that some cancer patients feel. It's all about money. Money isn't evil, but making money without being responsible and without genuinely looking out for the best interest of the patient is inexcusable. There are also a number of dishonest people in conventional medicine, but my primary purpose is to inform you of the best and the worst in the field of alternative medicine and nutrition so that you understand it fully from the beginning.

Chapter One—The Commandments of Nutrition, Supplements, and General Health—is an overall guide for the proper use of supplements. It is my sincere hope that once you have finished this book you will have a complete understanding of both nutrition and alternative medicine treatments for prostate cancer. Please pass this information along to your friends, sons, daughters, spouse, and co-workers so that as many people as possible can benefit from your under-standing.

Each chapter is divided into three sections—A, B, and C. Section A briefly explains the subject matter at hand. For instance, in the garlic chapter, Section A offers general information about garlic. Section B discusses the results of medical research on garlic in regard to treatment of prostate cancer, and Section C pro-vides specific recommendations for the use of garlic as either a preventive meas-ure or for treatment of prostate cancer.

Section C also provides information on the cost, dosage, and side effects of each chapter's topic. A "Bottom Line" is included at the end of each chapter with a "yes," "no," or "maybe" recommendation. I have included the "maybe" recommen-dation because sometimes there is not enough research data available to make a complete determination, although early results may look promising. Options that look promising should not, in my opinion, be kept from the public. Instead, you should have objective and unbiased information to help you make your decisions. Please let me stress that you must discuss these options with your doctor; other medical conditions or your medical history may not make you an ideal candidate for a particular alternative treatment.

The information provided in *The ABC's of Nutrition & Supplements for Prostate Cancer* is based on extensive research taken from many overall studies and other pertinent medical information. This book will enable you to take a giant step not only toward understanding nutrition and supplements, but—more importantly—taking more responsibility for your health.

Good Reading!
Mark Moyad, M.P.H.

1

The Commandments of Nutrition, Supplements, & General Health

The Commandments of Nutrition, Supplements, & General Health

These days everyone seems to be talking about which supplements to take to either prevent prostate cancer or stop it from progressing. Before we talk about what to take we must first understand the role of supplements and their safe and proper use. When taken incorrectly, the benefits of supplements can be lost, you may experience side effects, and you may not be getting your money's worth from the product(s).

The *Commandments of Nutrition and Supplements* are guidelines to help you make decisions about your health. If you study these commandments before you begin taking supplements you will possess far greater knowledge and experience greater success than the average consumer.

COMMANDMENTS OF NUTRITION AND SUPPLEMENTS

I. Regard Articles and Advertising About Supplements with Caution.

If you were to follow the advice given by all the self-proclaimed "experts"—or that found in supplement magazines—you could easily spend a good portion of your day and a good portion of your money consuming their products.

You need to be very careful before you decide which, if any, supplements you need. Why? Advertising for supplements is hard to regulate. Supplements do not require FDA approval, so the FDA cannot regulate the manner in which they are advertised, other than to prevent manufacturers from making specific claims about a product. Because of the manner in which a product is advertised, you may feel it is absolutely essential to your health. Let's look at one simple example: beta-carotene. If you were to visit my office and ask if you should take beta-carotene, for example, I could easily refer you to an article that indicates that people who take beta-carotene along with other supplements have a decreased risk of dying from cancer. On the other hand, if I didn't want to encourage you, I could refer you to studies that showed beta-carotene could increase your chance of getting lung cancer if you drink alcohol and smoke.

► Any time you are thinking about taking a supplement or changing your diet, make certain that you follow the advice of someone who has objectively reviewed all of the studies on the supplement, vitamin, or diet. You stand a far greater chance that the information you receive is sound, unbiased advice.

▶ Don't play the lottery game with your health. Supplements that have not been thoroughly tested in clinical trials are not safe for you to experiment with on your own. You are taking a very big chance with your health when you take a supplement based solely on hope.

▶ Immune boosters are not necessarily good for you. People immediately think that an immune booster provides a benefit. This is absolutely not true. The immune system is so large and complex that boosting the entire system or even the part you are specifically concerned about is not necessarily possible. There are thousands of products that boost the immune system but are worthless against cancer. Please, re-examine the effective cancer treatments available today: sur-gery, radiation, cryosurgery, hormone ablation, and chemotherapy. These treatments do not work by boosting the immune system, but instead by affecting a specific pathway of the disease and destroying tumors directly or removing them. Let's take a look at St. John's Wort and echinacea. Either may be potential partial immune boosters, but neither has been adequately tested against cancer. In some cases it is not a positive thing to boost an immune system that is already overexcited, e.g., in people with autoimmune diseases such as lupus or allergies. Your immune system may need to be suppressed or decreased. The medical profession is still trying to determine how best to use the immune system—primarily through the use of gene or vaccine therapies—in the fight against cancer.

II. Natural First and Supplement Second.

Why take beta-carotene, for example, when you can eat fruits and vegetables that contain not only beta-carotene but many other beneficial anticancer compounds as well? In this case it is better to find a natural source of beta-carotene than to take a supplement. (Please refer to Chapter 3—Beta-Carotene.)

Let's review one of my favorites, vitamin E. Vitamin E is very, very difficult to obtain from any natural source. Fatty nuts, margarine, and mayonnaise are natural sources of vitamin E. However, I cannot recommend any of these because they also contain a lot of fat. (As you will learn later in this book, fat and excess calories are not good for you in terms of prostate cancer.) In this case it makes sense to stay away from the natural source and take a vitamin E supplement. (Please refer to Chapter 18—Vitamin E.)

Once in a great while in the treatment of prostate cancer we come across something that can be consumed both naturally and in supplement form—for example, soy products. Soy is found naturally in soybeans, tofu, and soy milk. These sources of soy are all very helpful in fighting prostate cancer. Soy supplements in the form of soy protein powder (but not soy capsules or pills neccessarily are also good for you. The reason it is good to consume soy both naturally and as a supplement is that your body requires a tremendous amount if the soy is to have an effect against cancer. The recommended amount is so high that it is actually difficult to take too much. (Please refer to Chapter 8—Flaxseed and Soy.)

Fruits and vegetables are the best natural source of vitamins and minerals. Supplements should only be used when natural sources are difficult to obtain.

III. Moderation is Best.

Almost everything in life is better in moderation. If you eat too much fat you could be setting yourself up for heart disease or cancer. However, if you eat too little fat it could potentially create a number of other unhealthy situations.

Let's briefly review a few examples of moderation. Alcohol in moderation seems to increase your levels of HDL, or good cholesterol, while alcohol in large quantities can make your immune system suppressed or cause liver damage. How about driving a car? If you drive a car too fast you increase your chances of having an accident, while driving too slow can do the same thing. Driving at the recommended speed limit provides you with the greatest opportunity to complete your journey safely. What about sleep? If you sleep more than eight to ten hours a night, it could be a sign of depression and actually make you more tired during the day. Sleeping too little also makes you tired during the day.

Here's a quick review of a few popular supplements:

Vitamin C
Too little vitamin C provides little benefit for you, while too much vitamin C can act as a pro-oxidant and actually cause damage to the body.

Selenium
Too little selenium probably has no effect, while too much selenium can cause hair loss, nail disease, nausea, and diarrhea.

Vitamin D
Too little vitamin D prevents calcium from being absorbed by the body, while too much vitamin D can cause you to be hypercalcemic, absorbing too much calcium. If you absorb too much calcium it can be deposited in your blood vessels or organs, which is extremely harmful.

What about the sun? If you get too little sun exposure, your body responds by making only small amounts of vitamin D, and if you get too much sun you could be increasing your risk of skin damage and skin cancer.

The point? Too little or too much of anything is not good—everything in moderation is the best approach.

In terms of preventing prostate cancer, we now have a good idea of the appropriate level of moderation. Once you are diagnosed with cancer the definition of moderation is likely to change. You are no longer avoiding disease, but instead trying to prevent it from progressing. Levels of moderation for supplement use during radiation, chemotherapy, and surgery also remain undetermined, although we should have a better idea very soon.

In the second commandment we discussed the issue that few natural foods (fruits and vegetables) provide too much of anything, so you should feel free to eat them whenever you wish. (Just don't go overboard.) In cultures that regularly consume fruits and vegetables in large amounts, the level of moderation seems to be extremely high. The reality is that it isn't—people in the United States just aren't accustomed to consuming the same quantities and tend to believe quantities consumed in other cultures are very high. Green tea is a good example. Studies from Japan and China have shown that the benefit from green tea is not present unless you drink up to ten cups of green tea or more per day! Have you ever tried to drink ten cups of anything per day? It's tough. It's better to focus on making green tea a permanent part of your lifestyle by drinking one to several cups per day.

IV. Always Take Supplements During or Near Mealtime.

Almost all supplements should be taken with a meal or up to 20 to 30 minutes before or after meals. There are two simple reasons why. First, your body will absorb it better when it is taken with a meal. Vitamin E is a classic example: unless it is taken with food (or a small amount of fat), little to none of it is absorbed. Second, one of the most frequently cited reasons for not being able to tolerate a supplement is stomach upset. Selenium, taken on an empty stomach, can cause a lot of gas and stomach pain. This problem can be virtually eliminated in most cases if the supplement is taken at or close to mealtime. A few people always drop out of supplement trials early due to stomach or digestive problems. It is likely that many could have remained in the trial if the supplements had been taken with food. The two exceptions to this guideline are PC-SPES and essiac tea. (Refer to Chapter 11—PC SPES and Chapter 14—Tea.)

Unless otherwise instructed, take your supplements with a meal, please! In fact, as a constant reminder of this commandment, I leave my supplements in the middle of the dining room table to remind me not only to take them, but also to take them with a meal.

Whenever possible, take supplements with meals.

V. Start Low and Slowly Increase Your Dosage.

It is a common misconception that if a supplement is good for you it is even better if consumed in large quantities. Absolutely not! You need to allow your body to tolerate and adjust to supplements. Most medications start at a low dosage, and then if necessary the physician increases the dosage. It is no different with supplements. Let's say you need to take 800 International Units (IU) of vitamin E to control hot flashes. Begin with 200 IU, after a few weeks increase to 400 IU, after a few more weeks increase to 600 IU, and finally after a few more weeks increase to 800 IU. This gives your body time to adjust to the dosage. Your body is very complex—in some ways it is very strong, while in other ways it is a delicate machine. Give it a chance to become accustomed to a new supplement ritual.

Maybe you've already made the mistake of taking too much of a vitamin or supplement. What should you do? Just as your body needs a chance to become accustomed to a high dosage, it also needs a chance to adjust to a lower dosage. In the same way that you increase dosage, you can also decrease dosage.

Allow your body time to adjust to supplements—don't dramatically increase or decrease doses!

VI. Play It Safe—Take Only Those Supplements Proven Effective in Clinical Trials.

There remains a tremendous amount of information yet to review regarding nutrition and supplements. For now, it is best to take advantage of what we know for sure. Take the use of selenium as a treatment for prostate cancer, for example. In clinical trials, patients who took 200 micrograms (mcg) per day of selenium did very well. (Please refer to Chapter 12—Selenium.) Following this news, several supplement companies began manufacturing selenium at doses much higher than needed and with fancy additives such as zinc and a variety of herbs. This was done so that in marketing these supplements they could claim an overall healthful effect for the general population and therefore sell them to a larger segment of the market. The question is, Why would anyone take a chance on these products?

Play it safe and take only those supplements proven effective in clinical studies. Don't waste your money on supplements with fancy extras.

VII. Read the Label.

When studying supplements, one of your goals is very simple. You should never buy any supplement without first being able to adequately read the label and understand what you are purchasing. Many patients rely on a specific brand or a doctor's own supplement and have no idea what they are taking. It can be dangerous when a doctor recommends his or her own supplements.

Many patients purchase supplements without understanding how to read the ingredient label, thereby not knowing what they are taking. Take vitamin E, for example. You should understand all of the different types of vitamin E and be able to recognize which are made in the laboratory and which are taken from natural sources just by reading the labels. (Please refer to Chapter 18—Vitamin E.) You need to be able to read supplement labels to understand what you are purchasing. It's that simple. The next time someone recommends a supplement, stop, research and then make your decision. It's your health!

VIII. Do Not Expect Miracles Overnight—Patience and Commitment are Rewarded.

In general, people seem to believe that you can take a supplement for a few days and see an immediate result. This is rarely the case. Most supplements require a long-term commitment before any benefits are felt. Research clearly supports this. For example, women who took folate (from a multivitamin) reduced their chances of being diagnosed with colon cancer, but did not actually see this benefit until 15 years later. The same is true of another group of women who wanted to reduce their chances of cataracts by taking vitamin C—no benefit was observed until after 15 years. If you had followed these women for only five or ten years, it may have seemed as if very little benefit occurred from the use of either vitamin C or folate. However, after 15 years the benefits were huge.

Please remember that research indicates that when taking supplements you need to commit to their use over a long period of time. In all likelihood you will not see overnight results.

IX. Never Focus on One Single Aspect of Health.

Heart disease is the leading cause of death among men and women. In fact, men are eight to ten times more likely to die of heart disease than prostate cancer, and women are eight to ten times more likely to die of heart disease than breast cancer. Even after a man is diagnosed with prostate cancer, he is still more likely to die of another disease, especially heart disease. Why do I mention this? If you want to increase your chances of living a longer life you should focus on your overall health, not just the prevention of cancer. This is much easier said than done, but it is very, very important. The exception to this is, of course, is if you are in a life-threatening situation.

Here's an example. A 57-year-old man with localized prostate cancer decided on a treatment of hormonal shots in combination with seed implantation and external beam radiation. His chances of being disease-free in the next five to ten years were very good. However, for the ten years prior to his prostate cancer diagnosis he had also battled an extremely high cholesterol level. Once he began dealing with the prostate cancer he completely ignored his cholesterol level. His risk of a fatal heart attack was far greater than any other condition of his health. Today, he is watching his diet and taking supplements and medication for his cholesterol level—which is 100 points lower!

Focus on your overall health. It will greatly increase your chances of living longer.

X. Supplements Are Only a Piece of the Health Puzzle.

A recent study clearly demonstrated that in most cases men and women who take supplements regularly are also more likely to—among other things—exercise, avoid smoking and excess alcohol, keep stress to a minimum, and visit their doctors annually. Remember that if you want to have a long and healthy life, supplements and a nutritious diet are only small pieces of the puzzle.

The following few tips will help you along the way to a healthier life:

Exercise Regularly
Go to a health club and work out—take a friend!
Walk when you can. Use the steps—not the elevator—and park farther away from the mall, walk to church or to the market, etc.

Decrease Your Stress Level
Make an appointment for a massage or a facial, work in the garden, walk, or enjoy leisurely meals and meaningful conversation with good friends. Find out what works for you and do it!

Stay Mentally Healthy
Place more emphasis on your friendships and relationships. Good friends and family are very healthy for you. Surround yourself with people who are positive, happy, and supportive.

Control Your Weight
Weight is related to so many serious health problems—various cancers, high blood pressure, etc. Weight control is as important as taking supplements.

Be Aware of Your Attitude or Perspective

If you are surrounded by "negative energy" or extremely pessimistic individuals, maintain a distance. Healthy and happy relationships will help you remain healthier and happier.

Never Smoke

Enough said.

Eat Fruits and Vegetables

Incorporate a variety of fresh fruits and vegetables into your weekly diet.

Everything in Moderation

This includes alcohol, the sun, and supplements. Too much of anything is never good.

Never Have an Unhealthy Obsession with Health

I meet individuals on a daily basis who are completely consumed with what they should and shouldn't eat and drink. This is absolutely unhealthy behavior, both physically and mentally, for anyone. Be kind to yourself. You can correct past mistakes in your health while trying to extend your life, but please don't forget to cherish today. If you are eating healthy on a day-to-day basis you should be pleased with yourself. Here's what I want you to do: This is be kind to you day. Go out and buy yourself a big chocolate chip cookie (or whatever your favorite treat happens to be) and then go see a movie with a loved one.

Just about everyone has a story about someone they know who abused his or her body as much as they wanted and still lived a long and healthy life. Frequently I hear about someone who ate too much, drank too much, never exercised, smoked, and lived to be 90 years old or more. My own grandmother smoked, never exercised, and used lard for cooking every day, and she lived into her nineties! Just remember, though, for every individual who lived recklessly and survived to live a long life, there are at least ten individuals who didn't. Supplements are just one step in the right direction. Living a healthy lifestyle must also be a part of your daily activities. Oh, and reading this book is a good idea—odds are that if you do you will have a better grasp of healthy living.

XI. Store Your Supplements in a Cool, Dark, Dry Place.

In order to make sure that your supplements remain stable and do not expire early it is important to store them in the proper place. Never put them in the refrigerator—they will collect too much moisture. Never place them on top of the refrigerator either, it's too warm up there. Place them in a cupboard, in a medicine cabinet, or on top of the dining room or kitchen table, out of direct sunlight. I leave mine on the dining room table so that I remember not only to take them but also to take them with a meal.

When you travel, it is easy to take your supplements along in a small container. I've found that a film canister works very well; it's compact, dark and easy to put in a small travel bag.

XII. Divide Your Daily Dosage.

If, for example, you take 400 IU of vitamin E daily, divide the dosage into 200 IU early in the day and 200 IU late in the afternoon or early evening. Dividing your dosages will allow your body to tolerate the supplement better and reduce any side effects. It will also allow the supplement to remain in your bloodstream for 24 hours, thereby giving you the full benefit of the supplement. Either purchase smaller doses and take them twice per day or cut your pills in half. More than 250 to 500 mg of vitamin C taken at one time does not allow complete absorption— it is just eliminated from the body. If you are taking 200 mcg of selenium daily and experiencing stomach upset, try taking a 100 mcg tablet twice a day. It will reduce your chance of side effects dramatically and will keep the selenium in your bloodstream all day long.

XIII. Every Positive Has a Negative, and Vice Versa.

People tend to believe that there are no negative effects associated with nutrition and supplements. Unfortunately, most everything in life comes with some kind of "catch." If you are going to take supplements you need to understand the negatives as well as the positives. A popular misconception is that when buying organic fruits and vegetables there is no downside. Let's examine that carefully. Organic fruits and vegetables can be very expensive and you could find yourself spending a considerable amount of money to purchase them. This might be a negative for many people. Green teas are another example. Many contain caffeine, which we all know can keep you awake at night. Too much selenium can have serious side effects. The moral of the story: make certain you know what you are taking and what the side effects are.

XIV. Understand the Differences Between IU, mg, and mcg.

Dosages can be very confusing. Make sure you understand the dosage before you take any supplements. IU stands for International Units and is usually applied to fat-soluble vitamins, such as A, D, E, and K. An IU is a measure of the potency of a supplement and is very different from milligrams or micrograms. For example, 50 mg of vitamin E is not necessarily equal to 50 IU of vitamin E. It's actually closer to 75 IU in some cases. The abbreviation "mg" stands for milligrams, or one thousandth of a gram. The abbreviation "mcg" stands for microgram and is equal to one millionth of a gram. Many times patients tell me that they are taking 200 mg of selenium, for example, when they are truly only taking 200 mcg. Please take the time to understand the dosage levels. A mistake could have serious side effects.

IU = International Units
mg = milligrams (thousandths of a gram)
mcg = micrograms (millionths of a gram)

XV. Understand the Differences Between RDA, RDI, ODA, and ODI.

RDA—Recommended Daily Allowance.

The government established these allowances many years ago to represent dosages that may potentially eliminate your chances of contracting a rare nutritional disease. For example, 60 mg of vitamin C daily is the RDA to prevent diseases such as scurvy. Some, including me, believe that the current RDAs for the prevention of cancer, cancer treatment, and chronic diseases are too low.

RDI—Recommended Daily Intake.

These also have been established by the government and in some cases have recently replaced the RDAs. Please cross reference RDAs and RDIs, as they are not always the same. I believe that for the prevention and treatment of cancer the RDIs also are too low.

ODA—Optimum Daily Allowance.

This term is normally used to describe the maximum amount necessary to prevent a chronic disease. The ODA recommendations are usually much higher than the RDAs and RDIs.

ODI—Optimum Daily Intake.

This term is interchangeable with ODA, it is simply a matter of preference.

XVI. Natural vs. Synthetic Supplements.

There are supplement manufacturers who claim that natural supplements are better than synthetic vitamins. This, of course, allows them to raise the price, and at first sounds like it makes sense. Natural products must be better than anything created in a lab, right? Not so fast! The body is very good at differentiating between certain synthetic and natural supplements. Remember our friend vitamin E? The body seems to recognize natural vitamin E better than synthetic, but synthetic vitamin E has been used in the majority of the clinical trials. Vitamin C, on the other hand, is a different story. Natural vitamin C is not necessarily better than synthetic. Check the label and make sure whatever you purchase is pure product, i.e., pure vitamin C. You absolutely do not want to purchase anything with fillers, preservatives, or additives.

XVII. Organic Isn't Necessarily Better.

Organic fruits and vegetables—that is, those grown without pesticides or fertilizer—are not necessarily better for you than those from the supermarket. You should always wash your fruits and vegetables before you eat them to reduce the chemicals and pesticides that may be on their covering. The key is to purchase fresh fruits and vegetables, organic or not.

XVIII. Understand the Type of Study or Clinical Trial Used for Testing Supplements.

Supplements begin their lives in a test tube in a lab (in vitro). This, however, is only the first step in a long process. If a supplement shows promise in the lab, often manufacturers will advertise it as the new cure-all for everyone! This is very dangerous. There are literally thousands of supplements that, while arousing hope in the lab, prove to be worthless against disease.

After a successful lab study, the supplement is tested on animals (in vivo). If the results remain positive, a type of epidemiological (population) or clinical study can be performed. Once all of these tests are complete, a reasonable theory can be formed regarding the supplement's success.

Retrospective studies look back in time to determine what has worked. This is good, but it has its limitations. For instance, if I asked you what supplements you were taking in December of 1990, you might not be able to recall the information—hence the problem with retrospective studies. Patients are asked to recall their past history, which often creates an error called "recall error."

Prospective studies are much more powerful. In a prospective study a researcher follows a patient throughout the entire course of the study. Patients come in every few weeks or months to report what they are taking. It is much easier to follow dietary and supplement behaviors by recording things as they happen.

You should also familiarize yourself with the terms "placebo" and "blind study." Taber's Medical Dictionary defines placebo as an "inactive substance used in controlled studies of drugs/supplements." A placebo is given to one group of patients and the drug/supplement being tested is given to the other.

A blind study involves the use of a placebo group, but the people involved do not know if they are taking the supplement or a placebo. In a single-blind study the patients do not know who is taking which substance. The reason it is so important to conceal this information is very easy to understand. Perhaps you have decided to participate in a study on vitamin C and its effect on prostate cancer. You would most likely be very excited and hopeful about the possible results of the study. The excitement you feel may trigger your immune system, which in turn may temporarily alleviate your symptoms. It is important to researchers to observe both groups and study the final data without the patient's knowledge of whether he was taking a placebo or the supplement. This creates a more unbiased study.

If both the patients and researchers are unaware of who is taking the supplement and who is taking the placebo it is called a double-blind study. Why is this important? In some cases if a researcher knows who is getting the supplement and who is not, it may cause them to look more favorably on those who are taking the supplement. They may be subconsciously more attentive to improvements in the patient's condition. A double-blind, placebo-controlled study virtually eliminates the bias from both the patient's and the researcher's perspective. Everyone is treated equally and the results stand on their own merit.

Now that you understand all the terms, it's easier to understand, right? Remember, a prospective study allows a researcher to follow a patient from beginning to end of the test. (Note: Not all prospective studies are done in conjunction with a placebo group). Double-blind testing is when neither the patient nor the researcher knows who is taking the supplement and who is taking the placebo. Placebo-controlled means that a placebo is used in the study in conjunction with the supplement. Once a supplement has made it through lab, both in vitro (test tube) and in vivo (animal), and prospective, double-blind, placebo-controlled studies, you can be reasonably sure it works.

Occasionally in testing, discoveries are made serendipitously. Researchers are looking for one result and another—either good or bad—presents itself. For example, the study that found selenium effective in preventing prostate cancer was actually designed to determine whether selenium could prevent skin cancer.

test tube study (in vitro)
animal study (in vivo)
retrospective study (recall)
prospective study (follows the patient through the trial)

A prospective, double-blind, placebo-controlled study is very powerful—especially one that follows patients over a period of several years.

Keep in mind that this order can be reversed—but all of these studies should eventually be done before a recommendation is made about the effectiveness of a supplement.

XIX. Understand Why Your Doctor May Not Have as Much Knowledge About Nutrition and Supplements as About Conventional Medicine.

I am often asked why all doctors don't provide nutrition and supplement information to their patients. Most doctors want to provide their patients with this information, but they don't always know enough to thoroughly discuss these issues. For the most part it is because they were not provided these classes in medical school or residency. I received little to no information on this subject in medical school. I had to learn it from other sources, such as public health classes. In general, physicians want to learn more about the subject.

Every once in a while patients complain about a doctor who does not want to hear anything about the use of supplements and/or thinks they are worthless. My advice to you is simple. If you find a doctor who has no respect for your opinions, it is time to move on. Period! The doctor-patient relationship is bidirectional. The respect you show for your doctor's opinions and advice should be equal to the respect your doctor demonstrates for your thoughts, observations, and beliefs.

XX. Ask the Expert About Any Interest He or She May Have in a Supplement Company and Note Whether They Practice What They Preach!

If you ever listen to an expert speak on a health-related topic and he or she seems to push a product or supplement over and over again, ask if he or she has any financial interest or is involved with the company in any way. It's a good rule of thumb to research the speaker a little prior to attending a lecture or presentation. This is not meant to imply that if a financial interest in the product exists the speaker is not to be trusted. However, for an objective perspective it is important to understand all the circumstances before you make any commitment to a person or product.

In addition, if you are getting advice from a health professional, is it realistic? Do they practice what they preach? Is the person mentally and physically healthy? I believe this is important. Healthy behavior and practices can be addictive and infectious. If the person who gives you advice doesn't serve as a healthy role model it will be more difficult for you to follow their advice. Make sure your clinicians are taking care of themselves. In the long run they cannot provide you any long-term benefit if they aren't healthy enough to continue monitoring your health. The relationship between a health professional and a patient is like that of a family, and you want to ensure that it will be a lifelong relationship in both directions.

XXI. Every Antioxidant Can Also Act the Same as a Prooxidant.

To begin, here are a few definitions that may help you understand this commandment a little easier. An *antioxidant* is an agent that prevents or inhibits free radicals from being made, and a *prooxidant* is an agent that promotes free radical production. A *free radical* is a molecule which in some cases may damage the body. containing an odd number of electrons.

I wish we could take the word antioxidant out of circulation for a while. It's overused, and people don't understand that antioxidants can behave the same as prooxidants when taken incorrectly. While some antioxidants can stop free radicals and promote healing, in the wrong situation they encourage the production of free radicals and discourage healing. For example, lycopene is one of the most powerful antioxidants found in nature and may possess the ability to fight prostate cancer. However, in a number of laboratory studies, lycopene—taken as an individual supplement—has encouraged the growth of prostate tumors. What does this mean? Lycopene in its natural form, behaves as an antioxidant. When you remove lycopene from its natural environment it can behave as a prooxidant (or antioxidant) and may cause negative side effects. Remember Commandment II? Always look for a natural source first! If you are unable to locate a natural source or obtain the proper dosage, and the supplement is safe and effective, by all means use it. When taken in natural form, lycopene (found in fruits such as grapefruit, tomato, and watermelon), has been shown in tests to act as an antioxidant, thereby potentially reducing the risk of cancer. This does not mean that taken by itself as a supplement it will create the same effect. (Please refer to Chapter 10—Lycopene.)

XXII. The Differences Between Fat-Soluble and Water-Soluble Vitamins Can Be Minimal.

There are primarily four fat-soluble vitamins:
    Vitamin A
    Vitamin D
    Vitamin E
    Vitamin K

Fat-soluble means that the body normally stores them in large quantities. The more you take, the more you are likely to store these vitamins in your body in a substance such as fatty tissue.

Most of the remaining vitamins are water-soluble. Water-soluble means that the body does not normally store them in large quantities. The more you take, the more you are likely to eliminate them as waste.

Vitamin C is consumed in very large quantities by a tremendous number of people who believe their bodies will naturally eliminate any they do not need. However, vitamin C can create side effects, and if taken in very large doses it can act as a prooxidant. You should be just as careful when taking water-soluble vitamins as you are when taking fat-soluble vitamins. As far as research has shown, the only noticeable difference between fat-soluble and water-soluble vitamins is that fat-soluble vitamins require a little fat in your diet to be adequately absorbed.

XXIII. Never Choose a Favorite Fruit or Vegetable and Ignore All the Others.

Recently it was discovered that tomatoes reduce the risk of prostate cancer. This caused a great many people to begin eating them on a regular basis. The same studies indicated that a variety of other fruits and vegetables also reduced prostate cancer occurrence. (Please refer to Chapter 10—Lycopene.) The best plan is to eat a variety of fruits and vegetables in order to take advantage of the thousands of different anticancer compounds they contain. If you limit yourself to only one or two fruits or vegetables you miss out on everything else.

XXIV. Never Have an Unhealthy Obsession with Health and Supplements.

Recently, in the middle of a talk on breast cancer a young woman told me that she loves grapes but no longer eats them because they take too long to eat. I had to ask why. She explained that she had read that grapes retain pesticides in their skin, so in order to eat them she had to peel all their skins off and, well, it simply took too much time. This is the perfect example of an unhealthy obsession with health. Please don't misunderstand. I know it is extremely difficult when you have cancer not to be obsessed with your health, but I truly believe that at times people carry this so far that it becomes an additional source of stress, and thereby unhealthy. Eating right and supplementing has to be a stress-free adventure—if not, what is the point? Pesticides on grapes? Wash them before you eat them or buy organic grapes. You are taking such good care of yourself by eating fruits and vegetables instead of fatty or sugary foods—be happy! Unhealthy obsessions are an all too common occurrence.

Don't worry so much when you eat a little fat, sugar, or protein, or because you don't have the newest supplement on the market—worrying is unhealthy. The long-term consequences of worrying so much or becoming obsessed with your health are much worse for your condition than eating a sugar cookie or not taking the latest supplement. Remember, a healthy attitude is as much a part of your total overall health as eating right.

XXV. You Cannot Duplicate A Segment of Another Culture and Experience Total Transformation.

It is impossible to copy one aspect of healthy behavior from another culture and experience the same results. For example, simply drinking green tea because the Japanese do is not going to produce the same results. The consumption of green tea is only one aspect of their culture. The same study says that the more green tea you drink the less likely you are to smoke and the more likely to exercise, eat and drink soy products, and maintain a healthy weight. There are also those aspects of different cultures that are difficult to measure. Several years ago I spent time in both Austria and Singapore. People took breaks from work during the day, they ate meals peacefully, and were most certainly not on their cell phones screaming at the person in the next car while eating a bag of french fries for lunch. A healthy culture carries with it an almost infinite number of healthy behaviors, some measurable and some not measurable. It is important to look at your overall lifestyle, including your profession, relationships and hobbies, etc., as having an impact on your general health.

XXVI. Understand the Placebo Effect.

Sound crazy? Not really—it's easy to explain. The placebo effect is one of the strongest treatments in medicine and truly demonstrates that what the mind believes, the body will try to achieve. A placebo is a compound, pill, or procedure with no real medicinal value or benefit. However, some people become so excited or feel so much better simply because they are taking a pill or having a procedure performed that their condition actually improves. Let me cite a few examples. Men who have enlarged prostates (benign prostatic hyperplasia, or BPH) can be given a number of prescription drugs to treat their condition. In nearly all of the original clinical trials, up to one-third of the placebo group also experienced improvement in their symptoms. In the original Viagra studies about 25% of the men taking the placebo experienced stronger erections. In the original clinical trials for Propecia—an FDA-approved drug for hair loss and baldness—about 40% of men on placebo maintained their hair count and/or grew new hair.

These examples demonstrate that if the mind is truly convinced that something is possible, it just might happen! If you are taking a nonharmful substance or placebo, and it helps, then by all means continue to do so if at all possible.

XXVII. Stick With What You Know is Good for You—Don't Be Confused by Conflicting Information.

Exercise. We know that exercise is good for both your overall physical and mental health—though at times information surfaces that indicates it may not affect a specific area of your health. A recent study showed that women do not necessarily decrease their risk of breast cancer by exercising. Another study showed the same to be true of men who exercise to reduce their risk of prostate cancer. Yet many other studies have shown that exercise does aid in the prevention of cancer, especially breast and prostate cancer. We also know it can help reduce your risk of heart disease. What sense would it make to quit exercising when we are certain it provides many benefits?

XXVIII. You Do Have Control Over Your Health Regardless of Your Genetic History.

Based on my genetic history I am at increased risk for an aneurysm, high blood pressure, high cholesterol, skin cancer, and prostate cancer. Although my genetic history points to high risk for these conditions, I will never simply give in and wait for them to happen. Research shows that while genetics plays a role in cancer and heart disease we can still have a lot of control over our own health. In fact, even twins who have bad genetic histories have a lot of control over their own health! You are not doomed to live a shorter life because of your family history. If you take care of yourself you may never experience that which your ancestors did. In the case of high cholesterol, it may also be possible that your family members ate foods that caused their cholesterol to be high. If you maintain a low-cholesterol diet you may always have a normal cholesterol level.

Do the right thing—take care of yourself!

XXIX. Specific Dietary Recommendations Are Not Always Necessary or Realistic.

We live in a society that in many areas—including our health—exists from moment to moment. One minute we are committed to a certain exercise or supplement and the next minute we have abandoned it for something new. When salmon was reported to be of benefit for overall health it soon afterward became challenging to find at the market—absolutely everyone was eating salmon! The same thing happened when it was reported that tomatoes were beneficial for the prevention of prostate cancer.

We often make radical changes in our behaviors that are, at best, temporary. Look at all the different diet programs and reflect for a moment on how rapidly they change and how long most people stick to them. In issues related to health and disease it is very important to make changes in a conscious and permanent manner. Take a series of small steps and over time you will find that you have made a large change a permanent part of your life. Sudden or massive changes can be a little like New Year's resolutions. Every year on January 1st people resolve to make this next year different. The statistics of those who actually stick to their resolutions through February are grim.

I have never been a big fan of specific dietary recommendations that insist on such things as one specific cooking oil, specific vegetables and fruits, and dictates such as "never" and "always." Let's be realistic. We are not robots. Human behavior dictates our day-to-day lives, and as far as making a particular diet a part of our day-to-day routine—well, it's tough. Let's take a look at another example. The government released a campaign a few years back that said it was necessary to eat five servings of fruit and vegetables a day to reduce your risk of cancer. First, how many people actually know what "a serving" is? Secondly, does five servings a day mean it is okay to eat four servings of fruit and one serving of vegetables, or two servings of fruit and three servings of vegetables, or does it mean that you should eat five servings of fruit and another five servings of vegetables every day? It is very difficult to consistently eat five fruits and vegetables per day. It is more realistic to suggest that a variety of fruits and vegetables become a permanent part of your everyday diet.

Salmon has received a lot of positive focus lately, so people are in a salmon eating frenzy! Research has consistently shown that eating one serving of fish per week, whatever type, can reduce your chances of dying suddenly. Please note that individuals in this particular study consumed many types of fish, including: canned tuna, mackerel, salmon, sardines, bluefish, swordfish, shrimp, lobster and scallops—not just salmon. This makes a lot of sense. How long can you eat salmon before you never want to see a piece of it again for as long as you live? The point is not to be obsessed with the type of fish and serving amount, but simply to eat some fish every week. This is much easier to follow for an entire lifetime, it's realistic, and it's exactly what the research indicates is best for you. The next time you hear about the benefits of a food that is not currently a part of your diet, try to include it with the other foods you eat. The most important thing is to make certain you eat a variety of fruit or vegetables and other healthy foods every week, as opposed to one specific food over and over. Variety is the spice of life!

Added tip: include healthy behaviors with your meals, such as eating slowly while conversing with family or friends. Not only is it healthy, but you will very quickly find that you look forward to this time with your loved ones.

XXX. If You Are on Medication to Control a Condition, Remember That the Condition Still Exists—It Is Simply Controlled.

When cancer patients are asked if they have other health problems often they reply (for example), "No, but I take blood pressure medication." This is a little frightening. When a patient is taking medication to control a condition it simply means that, ideally, the condition is under control—it is not cured. It is temporarily being taken care of with medication. There is an inherent danger with some prescription medications in that frequently when they relieve symptoms, people think the condition is cured. What is in fact true is that these conditions may be a strong signal that you need to incorporate healthier behaviors into your life.

Please remember that your health is an ever-present challenge that depends on your perspective. When placed on prescriptions or diagnosed with a serious disease, people sometimes think, "Why me?" Others say, "Okay, I am going to beat this thing. This is my wakeup call that time on earth is not infinite and I need to live and love like tomorrow may never come." Which perspective do you think is healthier?

YOU ARE PRIMARILY RESPONSIBLE FOR YOUR HEALTH!

It is up to you! Keep track of your records, know your cholesterol level, blood pressure, etc. (actual values and numbers, not just normal or not normal). The more knowledge you have the more likely you are to take the right steps and make the right decisions toward a healthy and satisfying life.

2

Aspirin

In this chapter:

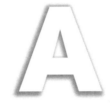

What is Aspirin?

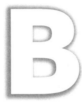

What the Medical Research Tells Us

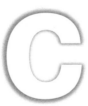

Bottom Line on Aspirin

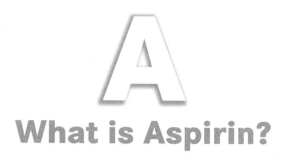

What is Aspirin?

"There is a bark of an English tree, which I have found by experience to be a powerful astringent, and very efficacious in curing anguish and intermittent disorders."
—The Reverend Mr. Edmund Stone of Chipping-Norton in Oxfordshire (April 25, 1763)

In 1757 the Reverend Stone tasted some willow bark, which was an already popular folk remedy, and decided to study it further. To his delight he discovered (from a small clinical trial he did with a few patients) that it took care of simple problems such as fever, aches, and pains. The willow tree is the source of salicin, which is the compound the Reverend Stone tasted. A derivative of salicin is aspirin.

Aspirin is officially classified as a NonSteroidal Antiinflammatory Drug ("NSAID"). It is the NSAIDs to which all others are compared and the most commonly used. Approximately 15% of the patients who cannot tolerate aspirin can benefit by using another NSAID. Several work better than aspirin and cause fewer side effects (mainly stomach problems), although they can be more expensive.

Common NSAID

acemetacin	prescription
acetylsalicylic acid (aspirin)	**over-the-counter**
apazone	prescription
benoxaprofen	prescription
carprofen	prescription
cinmetacin	prescription
clonixin	prescription
diclofenac	prescription
diflunisal	prescription
fenclofenac	prescription
fendosal	prescription
fenoprofen	prescription
feprazone	prescription
flufenamic acid	prescription

flunixin	prescription
flurbiprofen	prescription
ibuprofen (Advil, Motrin)	**over-the-counter**
indomethacin	prescription
indoprofen	prescription
isoxepac	prescription
isoxicam	prescription
kebuzone	prescription
ketoprofen	prescription
meclofenamate	prescription
mefenamic acid	prescription
mofebutazone	prescription
naproxen (Aleve)	**over-the-counter**
niflumic acid	prescription
phenylbutazone	prescription
piroxicam	prescription
pirprofen	prescription
salsalate	prescription
sulindac	prescription
suxibuzone	prescription
tenoxicam	prescription
tolfenamic acid	prescription
tolmetin	prescription
trimethazone	prescription
zomepirac	prescription

NSAIDs are commonly used for aches and pains such as arthritis, back pain, and headache. Additionally, aspirin is often used to prevent heart attacks.

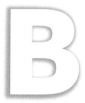

What the Medical Research Tells Us

Cells in the human body provide a compound that is converted into arachidonic acid (AA). Arachidonic acid is converted primarily into two compounds, but may go on to become a variety of other things.

Arachidonic acid can be converted into prostaglandins with the help of the enzymes COX-1 and COX-2. Prostaglandins aid in clotting or repairing a cut (inside or outside the body) and/or keeping the blood from becoming too thin. Often doctors advise patients to discontinue the use of aspirin and other NSAIDs prior to surgery to avoid the excessive bleeding that sometimes results from their use. In addition, aspirin can thin the blood to the point that it increases the chance of a hemorrhagic stroke or internal bleeding.

COX-1 helps maintain the body in a normal state. If you disturb COX-1 it can disrupt your normal body physiology. COX-2 causes inflammation in the body (which can also stimulate the growth of cancer). Aspirin can block COX-2, although not as well as it blocks COX-1.

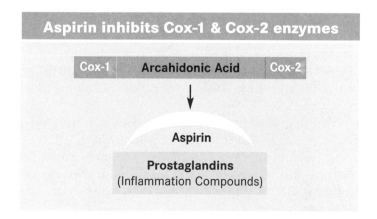

Lipoxygenase Inhibitors

The second conversion of arachidonic acid is via the lipoxygenase pathway. It creates "leukotrienes," which may cause inflammation and potentially increase cancer growth. Leukotrienes can make the airways in the lungs smaller (due to inflammation) so that it is difficult to breathe, sometimes resulting in asthma.

Prescribed Anticoagulants

There has also been a recent interest in the use of prescription anticoagulants for the treatment of prostate cancer. It is thought that cancerous tumors may need coagulation products to grow and move through the body. It is possible that if you eliminate these products from the blood cancer growth is inhibited. There have been a variety of prescription anticoagulant studies, for all types of cancer, that have shown promising results. Anticoagulants have slowed the progression of cancer and increased survival time for a number of patients. A great deal more research is needed to prove or disprove these theories.

Aspirin and other NSAIDs seem to behave in a fashion similar to prescription anticoagulant medications. It is an area in the treatment of prostate cancer that should be carefully monitored by anyone who is concerned.

Prostate Cancer

A number of studies have shown that prostate cancer may produce an increased amount of prostaglandins. These studies have also demonstrated the ability of NSAIDs to inhibit human prostate cancer cells.

Other studies, not entirely focused on prostate cancer, have shown limited reduction of cancer with the use of aspirin. A recent New Zealand study shed light on the possibility of using NSAIDs to reduce not only prostate cancer but also to retard its growth from localized to advanced stages. The men in the study who took NSAIDs or aspirin in low dosages (approximately 100 to 150 mg/day) were less likely to be diagnosed with advanced prostate cancer. Although the results of this study did not reach statistical significance, they pointed toward a decrease. It is possible that NSAIDs, including aspirin, inhibit the growth of more aggressive prostate cancers but do little to stop slower-growing cancers. Further research is being conducted.

How does aspirin help with prostate cancer? Once in the body, aspirin travels to the liver. There it is converted to, among other things, Salicylic acid. Salicylic acid has been shown, in the laboratory, to inhibit prostate cancer growth.

The production of prostaglandins (which may stimulate cancer growth) may also be inhibited by aspirin and/or other NSAID, thereby preventing the progression of prostate cancer.

COX-2 Inhibitors

"Cox-2 inhibitors" were introduced in 1999. These drugs are unique because they block only the COX-2 enzyme. They may be stronger than aspirin and other NSAIDs but produce fewer side effects. Currently they are primarily used for certain types of arthritis (i.e. osteoarthritis), but may prove effective in the future for cancer treatment.

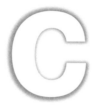

Bottom Line on Aspirin

Cost—Inexpensive

For less than $10 you can buy a month's supply.

Dosage and Type—30 to 325 mg/day

The dosage for other NSAIDs may differ—please talk to your doctor prior to the use of NSAIDs.

Researchers have agreed that 30 mg of aspirin is an effective dose to block prostaglandins. Regular aspirin/325 mg. Children's aspirin/81 mg. If you are taking aspirin to treat prostate cancer, try taking baby aspirin. It produces far less side effects.

If you do not tolerate aspirin well, try an enteric-coated aspirin taken with a meal. If you cannot tolerate any aspirin, talk to your doctor about another NSAID that does not cause the same side effects.

Acetaminophen products do not work the same as the NSAIDs. Therefore, nothing is known regarding their effect on cancer. Researchers are currently combining acetaminophen with NSAIDs in the laboratory to study its effect on various cancers. The early results are promising but much more research is needed. Pay close attention to future research in this area.

Side Effects—Hemorrhagic Stroke (Internal Bleeding), Ulcers, and Stomach Upset

Aspirin can cause hemorrhagic stroke and/or ulcers if taken in high doses for a long period of time. It can also cause you to bleed for a longer period of time. If you are scheduled for surgery, discontinue the use of aspirin one to two weeks prior to the surgery. If you take prescription blood thinners, aspirin may cause excessively thin blood.

If you cannot tolerate aspirin try an enteric-coated aspirin or an alternate NSAID. Always take with plenty of fluids and a meal to avoid side effects.

The Bottom Line
For the Prevention or Recurrence of Prostate Cancer—NO
For Localized Prostate Cancer—MAYBE
For Advanced Prostate Cancer—NO

Pay close attention to future research in this area of prostate cancer treatment. Discuss any concerns or questions with your doctor.

3

Beta-Carotene & Vitamin A

In this chapter:

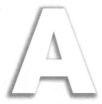

What are Beta-Carotene and Vitamin A?

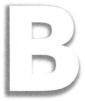

What the Medical Research Tells Us

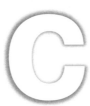

Bottom Line on Beta-Carotene and Vitamin A

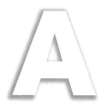

What are Beta-Carotene and Vitamin A?

Beta-Carotene

Carotenoids are antioxidants that play an important role in helping prevent various diseases, including some cancers. They are one of a group of pigments (organic coloring matter in the body), ranging in color from light yellow to red. The most commonly recognized is beta-carotene, which is found in carrots, but other carotenoids include lycopene (found in tomatoes) and lutein (found in spinach).

Carotenoids are commonly found in foods such as carrots, tomatoes, and spinach.

Carotene is a yellow pigment found in both plant and animal tissue. It is abundant in yellow vegetables, such as, carrots, squash, and corn. Carotene exists in several forms and is the precursor (a substance that precedes another substance) of vitamin A. It is stored and converted to vitamin A in the liver. Carotenes are the largest and most diverse group of pigments found in the world. They are fat-soluble, which, as we know from Chapter 1, means they are released, absorbed, and transported by fat in your diet and are not easily released into urine. Bile in the small intestines and food aid in the absorption of carotenes. If taken in large quantities they can be stored in the liver or fatty (adipose) tissue.

Carotene is found in carrots, squash, and corn.

Beta-carotene is only one of 600 carotenoids thus far discovered through research. It is an antioxidant that minimizes the damage caused by free radicals. Ingestion of large doses of vitamin A or Beta-Carotene supplements may cause of variety of toxic changes in the body.

Carotenoids are divided into two groups—those that can be converted into vitamin A and those that cannot.

Common carotenoids that can be converted to vitamin A after eaten: (5 to 10% of all known carotenoids):

alpha-carotene—red peppers
beta-carotene—carrots
cryptoxanthin—oranges

Common non-vitamin-A-forming carotenoids (90 to 95% of all known carotenoids):

lutein—spinach
lycopene—tomatoes

Beta-Carotene Facts

► Beta-carotene is one of the carotenoids that can be partially converted into vitamin A.

► Beta-carotene is converted in the intestines to a type of vitamin A known as retinol. This conversion is not particularly efficient—only 16 to 17% of all the beta-carotene you consume is converted.

► Beta-carotene in supplement form is normally sold in milligrams (mg) or International Units (IU).

► The greater the intensity of color in the fruit or vegetable, the higher the amount of beta-carotene it contains. Look for bright orange carrots, for example, to be sure you are purchasing those with high levels of beta-carotene.

Vitamin A

Vitamin A was the first fat-soluble vitamin discovered. Hence the "A" in vitamin A. It is formed in the body from precursors—yellow pigments of plants (alpha, beta, and gamma carotene). It is essential for normal growth and development, the normal function and integrity of epithelial tissue (cells that form the outer surface of the body and line the body cavities and prin-

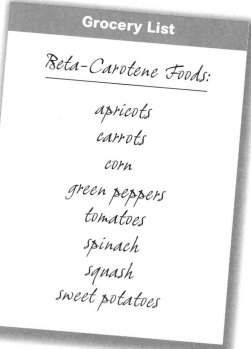

Grocery List

Beta-Carotene Foods:

apricots
carrots
corn
green peppers
tomatoes
spinach
squash
sweet potatoes

ciple tubes and passageways leading to the exterior), and normal tooth and bone development.

Vitamin A Facts

▶ Vitamin A supplements are normally sold in International Units (IU).
▶ Vitamin A was the first fat-soluble vitamin discovered.
▶ Vitamin A is stored in the liver.

Vitamin A in Common Foods (per 3.5-ounce (100-gram) Serving)

Food	Vitamin A
beef liver	44,000 IU
calf liver	22,500 IU
chili peppers	21,500 IU
chicken liver	12,000 IU
carrots	11,000 IU
dried apricots	11,000 IU
collard greens	9,500 IU
kale	9,000 IU
sweet potatoes	9,000 IU
parsley	8,500 IU
spinach	8,000 IU
mangoes	5,000 IU
squash	4,500 IU
cantaloupe	3,500 IU
apricots	2,500 IU
broccoli	2,500 IU

As you can see from the nutrition chart, beef, calf, and chicken liver contain large amounts of vitamin A. This shouldn't come as a complete surprise, since we know vitamin A is generally stored in the liver. You can also find it in relatively large amounts in some fruits and vegetables. Try to obtain vitamin A from natural sources rather than from supplements.

Retinoids

I mention retinoids at this point only to let you know of their existence and offer a brief explanation, although at this time I would not recommend their use. Here's why: retinoids are a class of compounds that include vitamin A. For instance, 4-HPR (also known as 4-hydroxyphenyl retinamide—a retinoid) is derived from vitamin A and has been successful in preventing some prostate tumors in animals. Retinoids warrant careful attention over the next few years. They are currently associated with quite a few side effects—such as headaches, skin, liver and vision problems—but may develop as a viable option within a short period of time if these side effects can be reduced.

What the Medical Research Tells Us

Beta-Carotene

We know from medical research that:

▶ Foods rich in beta-carotene and vitamin A are good for you.
▶ The supplement form of beta-carotene and/or vitamin A accomplishes little.

A 1993 New England Journal of Medicine study pointed out that the risk of heart disease is lower when beta-carotene is consumed from natural or dietary sources. In fact, even among male smokers who also had a high dietary intake of beta-carotene, there was a 30% decreased risk of heart disease.

In a related study, a group of 22,071 male physicians were followed for 12 years. Approximately half of these men took a 50-mg beta-carotene supplement every other day, while the other half took a placebo. The results were eye-opening: after 12 years of beta-carotene supplements there was no visible benefit proven in terms of incidence of malignant neoplasms, cardiovascular disease, or death from all causes. (Taber's Medical Dictionary defines neoplasm as "a new and abnormal formation of tissue, such as a tumor or growth." A neoplasm grows at the expense of healthy tissue).

No real benefit was found after taking beta-carotene supplements for twelve years.

Critics of this study claim that the dosage was insignificant and therefore prevented positive results. However, there is currently no evidence available supporting the use of beta-carotene supplements; therefore simply recommending a higher dosage would not be in anyone's best interest.

Two additional large clinical trials should be noted. Both found an increase in the risk of lung cancer among male smokers who took beta-carotene in supplement form.

Why then do you still hear good news about beta-carotene supplements? There have been a couple of studies in which beta-carotene supplements have been of some benefit. For example, beta-carotene was found to be of minimal benefit among women smokers who were at risk of cervical cancer and took 30 mg of beta-carotene daily for approximately six months. Another study, done in Linxian, China, showed that after taking beta-carotene (among other) supplements for five years there was an almost 10% decrease in overall deaths, a 13% decrease in death from cancer, and a 21% decrease in death from stomach cancer. Many beta-carotene supplement advocates use this trial to convince you that you should take beta-carotene. Please remember that neither group in these studies was comprised of particularly healthy individuals. Supplements often initially show better results with those who are undernourished or unhealthy, although it has not been proven that they provide any long-term benefits.

What does all of this mean? The bad news is that when it was discovered that in its natural form beta-carotene decreased the risk of cancer, researchers became hopeful that a supplement could be substituted for the same effect. Great idea, but the overall results for supplements have been disappointing.

The good news? Population studies have shown that increased consumption of foods rich in beta-carotene have been associated with a lower risk of many cancers. In two large recent clinical studies there was an increased risk of lung cancer with the use of beta-carotene supplements; however, it was found that among the individuals who began the study with high levels of natural beta-carotene in their blood, there was actually a lower risk of lung cancer! Don't fool yourself into thinking that a supplement can replace all the benefits of beta-carotene. Fruits and vegetables rich in beta-carotene are your best choice and provide many, many health benefits.

Vitamin A

Ditto! Foods rich in vitamin A provide you with a number of antioxidants and other potential anticancer compounds. Some experts will argue that you need vitamin A in supplement form because it can prevent certain eye diseases. This is only true if you rarely eat food containing vitamin A. Eye problems caused by a lack of vitamin A are a rare condition in the United States. Just remember to eat fruits and vegetables on a daily basis—and relax—you'll be getting plenty of beta-carotene and vitamin A.

Beta-Carotene, Vitamin A, and Prostate Cancer

The general conclusion from more than 3500 studies on beta-carotene points to a chance of reducing prostate cancer if you eat a diet low in fat and high in vitamin-rich fruits and vegetables.

Let's examine the effects of beta-carotene—in both natural and supplement form—on prostate cancer.

A closer look at the results of a beta-carotene trial among Finnish male smokers showed that taking a 20-mg beta-carotene supplement daily increased their risk of getting prostate cancer by 23% and of dying from prostate cancer by approximately 15%.

No benefit for reducing prostate cancer has ever been shown through the use of beta-carotene supplements!

Since 1981 there have been a number of studies that suggest that individuals who consume large quantities of food rich in beta-carotene may decrease their risk of cancer.

How? Men who consume beta-carotene from fruits and vegetables also seem to eat less fat. It may be that eating fruits and vegetables is an indicator of a healthier overall lifestyle that reduces the risk of prostate cancer. One of my favorite studies, published in 1988, examined the low amount of prostate cancer in Japan and concluded that one of the reasons for this was that Japanese tend to eat less meat (fat) and more fruits and vegetables. Fabulous conclusion! Many other studies have shown that as a person increases his consumption of fat, he also decreases his consumption of fruits and vegetables.

It's the same with Vitamin A. Supplements are not as beneficial for you as dietary sources. Additionally, the majority of population studies done on vitamin A supplements show that it does not lower your risk of prostate cancer. In fact, several studies have shown that the intake of vitamin A from meats can increase your risk of prostate cancer. How can this be? Vitamin A that is converted from natural beta-carotene comes from plants. As we have already learned, the more plant foods you eat, the lower your risk of prostate cancer. Vitamin A from meats, which are high in fat, increases your risk of prostate cancer. (Please refer to Chapter 7— Fat, Fatty Acids, and Fiber.) In Japan and several other areas of the world with a lower prostate cancer incidence, the main source of vitamin A is from vegetables.

In high prostate cancer risk areas, like the United States, the main source of vitamin A is from animal fats or meats. We can conclude that results of studies indicating a greater increase in prostate cancer along with the higher consumption of vitamin A are probably due to an increased intake of animal fat by these individuals.

It is best to obtain your beta-carotene and vitamin A from dietary sources of fruits and vegetables, such as green leafy vegetables, sweet potatoes, mangoes, and cantaloupes.

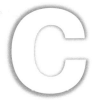

Bottom Line on Beta-Carotene and Vitamin A

Cost—Inexpensive
Cost of fruits and vegetables varies, however the benefits far outweigh their cost.

Dosage and Type
Once again, please do your best to consume both beta-carotene and vitamin A from dietary sources, mainly fruits and vegetables. I do not recommend specific amounts of each particular fruit or vegetable. It is more important that you incorporate the consumption of these healthy foods into your daily food plan. Choose fruits and vegetables and portions of each so that they become a permanent part of your diet.

Side Effects
Carotenemia (temporary skin discoloration), and increased risk of birth defects for pregnant women (in large dosages—more than 10,000 I.U./day)

As a general rule, beta-carotene can be taken for a long time before any side effects are seen. In fact, the only real problem with too much beta-carotene (from dietary sources) is a condition called carotenemia. This simply means that your skin may turn a slight orange color when you have too much in your system. It is harmless and it goes away after you discontinue use. Among individuals who are sensitive to the sun and burn easily this actually may provide some benefit. Pregnant women should not take vitamin A as a supplement; it has been shown to increase the risk of birth defects.

Food for Thought

Don't spend your money on supplements. Buy fruit and vegetables instead. Think about this: If you purchase these supplements at $10 a month for 5 years it will cost you $600, for 10 years—$1200, and for 15 years—$1800!

Take the money you save and go out for dinner (make sure you order some fruits and vegetables), see a movie, take a cooking class, get a massage, plan a vacation, buy someone you love flowers.

Beta-Carotene and Vitamin A Supplements—The Bottom Line

For Prevention or Recurrence of Prostate Cancer—NO
For Localized Prostate Cancer—NO
For Advanced Prostate Cancer—NO

Make sure you obtain plenty of both beta-carotene and vitamin A from dietary sources in your daily food intake plan. You can achieve this result by eating a variety of fruits and vegetables. Neither beta-carotene nor vitamin A in individual supplement form have been proven to reduce your chances of prostate cancer or to prevent it from progressing.

4

B Vitamins & IP-6

In this chapter:

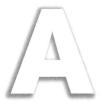

What are B Vitamins & IP-6?

What the Medical Research Tells Us

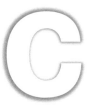

Bottom Line on B Vitamins & IP-6

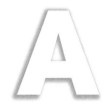

What are B Vitamins and IP-6?

B-Vitamins

B-vitamins are a group of water-soluble vitamins isolated from liver, yeast, and other sources.

B-vitamins are commonly known as:
B-complex vitamins
multiple B-vitamins
stress vitamins
B-50 vitamins
B-100 vitamins

B-vitamins refer to a much larger group of vitamins:
B1—thiamin
B2—riboflavin
B3—niacin and niacinamide or inositol hexaniacinate (no-flush niacin)
B5—pantothenic acid and pantethine
B6—pyridoxine
B12—cobalamin
folic acid or folate
biotin
choline
inositol
PABA (para-aminobenzoic acid)

▶ Thiamin, or B1, was the first B-vitamin discovered. It is important in carbohydrate metabolism and normal functioning of nervous tissue.

▶ Riboflavin, or B2, is vital to protein metabolism and normal growth, and is believed to aid in the relief of migraine headaches. It is B2 that causes the fluorescent yellow color to appear in urine.

►Niacin, or B3, and pantothenic acid, or B5, have been used in excess of 25 years to treat high cholesterol.

►Pyridoxine, or B6, is said to help with carpal tunnel syndrome and MSG sensitivity caused by various Chinese foods.

►B12, folic acid, and B6 may all help reduce the risk of heart disease by reducing blood levels of homocysteine, an abnormal by-product of amino acid metabolism.

These vitamins each play a unique role in the body and share similar properties. Many of these vitamins are found in the same foods and work together in the body. B-vitamins are popular because they give us energy and are needed for the proper metabolism of sugars (carbohydrates), fats, and proteins. During periods of stress the body loses vitamin B. It is most important to make certain you obtain enough vitamin B during stressful periods in your life. Finally, vitamin B helps reduce high levels of homocysteine (an amino acid), which may increase your risk of a heart attack, and may be involved in reducing a number of cancers.

Over the past few years, four of the B-vitamins have received a lot of attention as a result of their ability to reduce heart disease and, potentially, cancer. The "fabulous four" are B3, B6, B12, and folic acid. Each is easily obtained through dietary food sources.

Niacin Foods (B3)	milligrams (mg) per 3.5-ounce (or 100-gram) Serving
brewer's yeast	38
rice bran	30
wheat bran	21
peanuts	16
wild rice	6
sesame seeds	5
sunflower seeds	5
brown rice	5
pine nuts	5
red chili peppers	5
whole wheat grain or flour	4
wheat germ	4
barley	4
almonds	4
peas	3

Vitamin B6 Foods	milligrams (mg) per 3.5-ounce (or 100-gram) Serving
brewer's yeast	3
sunflower seeds	1
wheat germ	1
soybeans	0.8
walnuts	0.7
lentils	0.6
lima beans	0.6
black-eyed peas	0.6
navy beans	0.6
brown rice	0.6
hazelnuts	0.5
garbanzo beans	0.5
pinto beans	0.5
bananas	0.5
avocados	0.4
whole wheat flour	0.3
chestnuts	0.3
kale	0.3
spinach	0.3
turnip greens	0.3
sweet peppers	0.3
potatoes	0.3
prunes	0.2
raisins	0.2
brussels sprouts	0.2
barley	0.2
sweet potatoes	0.2
cauliflower	0.2

Vitamin B12 Foods	micrograms (mcg) per 3.5-ounce (or 100-gram) Serving
liver	25–100
clams	98
kidneys (lamb or beef)	30–60
oysters	18
sardines	17
trout	5

salmon	4
tuna	3
lamb	2
eggs	2
cheese	1–2
other types of fish	1

Folic Acid Foods	micrograms (mcg) per 3.5-ounce (or 100-gram) Serving
brewer's yeast	2,000
black-eyed peas	440
soy beans and soy flour	225–425
beef liver	300
wheat bran	200
beans (kidney, lima, navy)	125–200
asparagus	110
lentils	105
walnuts	80
spinach	80
kale	70
peanuts	60
broccoli	50
barley	50
peas	50
brussels sprouts	50
almonds	50
oatmeal	30
cabbage	30
figs	30
avocados	30
green beans	30
corn	30
coconuts	30
pecans	30
mushrooms	30
dates	30
blackberries	10
oranges	10

NATURAL SOURCES OF THE REMAINING B-VITAMINS:

Food	B1 milligrams (mg) per 3.5-ounce (100-gram) Serving
brewer's yeast	15.6
wheat germ	2.0
sunflower seeds	2.0
pine nuts	1.3
peanuts	1.1
soybeans	1.1
pecans	0.85
pinto beans and red beans	0.85
split peas	0.75
wheat bran	0.70
pistachio nuts	0.65
navy beans	0.65
oatmeal	0.60
whole wheat flour or grain	0.55
lima beans	0.50
hazelnuts	0.46
wild rice	0.45
cashews	0.45
mung beans	0.40
lentils	0.35
green peas	0.35
brown rice	0.35
walnuts	0.35
garbanzo beans	0.30
garlic	0.25
almonds	0.25
lima beans	0.25
pumpkin seeds	0.25
red chili peppers	0.20

Food	B2 milligrams (mg) per 3.5-ounce (100-gram) Serving
brewer's yeast	4.3
liver	2.7
almonds	.90

wheat germ	0.70
wild rice	0.65
mushrooms	0.45
red peppers	0.35
soy flour	0.35
wheat bran	0.35
collard greens	0.30
soybeans	0.30
split peas	0.30
kale	0.25
parsley	0.25
cashews	0.25
rice bran	0.25
broccoli	0.25
pine nuts	0.25
sunflower seeds	0.25
navy beans	0.20
beets	0.20
lentils	0.20
prunes	0.20
mung beans	0.20
pinto beans and red beans	0.20
black-eyed peas	0.20

B2 is also known as "Riboflavin."

Food	B5 milligrams (mg) per 3.5-ounce (100-gram) Serving
brewer's yeast	12.0
liver	8.0
peanuts	3.0
mushrooms	2.0
soybean flour	2.0
peas	2.0
pecans	1.5
soybeans	1.5
oatmeal	1.5
sunflower seeds	1.5
lentils	1.5

cashews	1.5
garbanzo beans	1.0
wheat germ	1.0
broccoli	1.0
brown rice	1.0
whole wheat flour	1.0
red chili peppers	1.0
avocados	1.0
black-eyed peas	1.0
wild rice	1.0
cauliflower	1.0
kale	1.0

B5 is also known as "Pantothenic Acid."

Biotin, a B-vitamin, is found in eggs (amount varies), cheese (amount varies), and many other foods. (The following foods contain such small quantities of biotin that it is listed as mcg, or micrograms.)

Food	Biotin micrograms (mcg) Per 3.5 Ounce (100 gram) Serving
brewer's yeast	200
liver	95
soy flour	70
soybeans	60
rice bran	60
peanut butter	40
walnuts	35
peanuts	35
barley	30
pecans	25
oatmeal	25
black-eyed peas	20
peas	20
almonds	20
cauliflower	15
mushrooms	15
lentils	15
brown rice	0

Choline, another B-vitamin, is used to manufacture acetylcholine, an important compound for memory and other functions. Lecithin, a precursor of choline, may fight cholesterol and depression, among other things.

Foods	Choline (and Lecithin)
Amount (♥ ♥ ♥ = > 100 milligrams, ♥ ♥ = 10–100 milligrams, ♥ = < 10 milligrams)	
liver (3.5 ounce)	♥ ♥ ♥
eggs (one)	♥ ♥ ♥
lecithin supplement (1 tablespoon, 7.5 grams)	♥ ♥ ♥
steak (3.5 ounce)	♥ ♥
peanuts (1 ounce)	♥ ♥
peanut butter (2 tablespoons)	♥ ♥
cauliflower (1/2 cup)	♥ ♥
coffee (6 ounces)	♥ ♥
orange (one)	♥ ♥
potato (one)	♥
milk (whole, 1 cup)	♥
grape juice (6 ounces)	♥
lettuce (1 ounce)	♥
tomato (one)	♥
apple (one)	♥
banana (one)	♥
whole wheat bread (1 slice)	♥
cucumber (1/2 cup)	♥
butter (1 teaspoon)	♥
ginger ale (12 ounces)	♥
margarine (1 teaspoon)	♥
corn oil (1 tablespoon)	♥

Inositol, again a B-vitamin, is most commonly found in fiber as phytic acid or inositol phosphate (IP6). When fiber enters the intestines, bacteria causes inositol to separate from phytic acid. Inositol is found naturally in:

animal foods (meats)
fruits
grains
nuts

seeds
legumes

PABA (para-aminobenzoic acid) is a member of the B-vitamin family that aids in the formation of folic acid and protein metabolism. It is often found in sunscreen because it protects against sunburn when applied to the skin (but not when taken orally). It is found in:

brewer's yeast
liver
kidney
grains
molasses

Vitamin B Facts

▶ Continued cooking over high heat or slow cooking destroys vitamin B.

▶ Vitamin B is water-soluble and is sold in milligrams or micrograms.

▶ Prolonged use of antibiotics may destroy the intestinal bacteria that normally produces some of the B-vitamins.

▶ Vitamin B helps reduce the risk of heart attack by reducing the levels of homocysteine (an amino acid) in the blood.

IP6

IP6, also known as phytic acid or inositol hexaphosphate, is a naturally occurring sugar or carbohydrate typically found in whole grains and high-fiber foods such as legumes and cereals. As a part of the vitamin B complex it has received much attention. IP1, IP2, IP3, IP4, and IP5 are also different types of inositol. Each can be found in nearly every cell in the human body.

Food	Quantity	IP6 Amount in milligrams (mg)
corn	1/2 cup	650
sesame seeds	3/4 cup	530
wheat bran	1-3/4 cups	460
beans	1/2 cup	250
brown rice	1/2 cup uncooked	220
corn bread	3-1/2 ounces	130

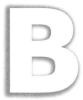

What the Medical Research Tells Us

B-Vitamins

Since there is little argument from doctors that pregnant women should take folic acid or folate to prevent certain birth defects, B-vitamins have become an essential aspect of prenatal health. However, B-vitamins play a much larger role than for prenatal care alone.

B-Vitamins and Cancer

Folic acid is important for maintaining methionine (an amino acid), which is paramount to the proper formation of DNA. If enough folate is not present in the body, potential problems in the formation of DNA can occur which in turn can lead to cancer. Several studies, including two male population studies, showed that an inadequate amount of folic acid might increase the risk of colon cancer. An even earlier study on women found a lower risk of colon cancer among women who obtained folic acid from a multivitamin. Four other case control studies have shown an increase in colon cancer among individuals with lower folic acid intake.

Cancer and Too Many B-Vitamins

B-vitamins are essential to the proper formation of DNA in nearly every cell. Overdosing with B-vitamins creates the potential situation of fueling cancerous cells with the material they need for creating more cancer cells. This has been shown to happen in both laboratory and animal studies. For example, thiamin (B1) supplies cells—cancerous or not—with more DNA. A recent paper urged patients that in order to be safe their daily dosage should not exceed more than 1.2 mg of thiamine, which is approximately the amount contained in a multivitamin. Overdosing with other B vitamins may potentially create the same harmful situation.

B-vitamin supplements in excess are not good if you have been diagnosed with cancer or are at high risk for cancer.

B-Vitamins and Prostate Cancer

Unfortunately, there have been very few studies on the effect of B vitamins and prostate cancer. Of the studies that have been done, a few have shown interesting results. One dietary study showed that men who either ate foods that contained vitamin B6 and/or took supplements with B6 had a slight decrease in prostate cancer risk. One theory for this is that B6 prevents the prostate from absorbing excessive amounts of hormones while the opposite is true when too little B6 is obtained. Another theory is that eating healthy foods, such as soybeans and other vegetables and fruits that contain B6—provides additional protective nutrients. Lastly, by eating healthy foods in larger quantities you are hopefully eating less fat, which again reduces the risk of prostate cancer. (Please refer to Chapter 7—Fat, Fatty Acid, and Fiber.)

An interesting study in 1987 showed that men who consumed a good amount of both B1 and B2 from dietary sources had a lower risk of being diagnosed with prostate cancer. Now, let me caution you that this was only one small study and it was done more than ten years ago. To date, B-vitamins for the treatment of prostate cancer have received little attention overall.

IP6

IP6 has been proven to promote cell differentiation (maintenance of healthy cells) in colon, prostate, and breast cancer tissue in the laboratory. In several laboratory and animal studies IP6 has demonstrated potential to decrease the growth of certain cancers. How? Researchers aren't sure exactly, but since IP6 contains a few properties similar to those of chemotherapy drugs, it is possible that it works in a similar way. It may also block certain sites that help cancers grow and may interact with iron and other potential free radicals to neutralize them and prevent them from increasing cancer growth. Please keep in mind at this point that although the early results are exciting they are from animal studies only. Presently, we don't know if IP6 will have any effect on the human body.

Recently IP6 has garnered a great deal of attention among prostate cancer patients and their health care providers. This is due to several reasons. First, people are now learning of the promising animal laboratory studies. This always offers the hope that throughout the remainder of trials results will remain positive. Secondly, IP6 is available commercially and is heavily advertised. In addition, in a laboratory study using human hormone-insensitive (refractory) prostate cancer cells, IP6 was able to inhibit the growth of some of these cells.

The bottom line is that IP6 has only been tested in the lab, on animals. You may recall that in Chapter 1, Commandment XVIII explained that animal testing is only the first phase of testing. There are many more tests yet to be completed, and any number of results—both good and bad—could be found. There is currently no solid evidence that this supplement works for men who have been diagnosed with or are trying to prevent prostate cancer. In addition, the supplement may interfere with the body's absorption of minerals. Let's proceed cautiously until we can review additional clinical data indicating that it works for the treatment of prostate cancer.

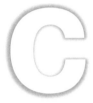

Bottom Line on B-Vitamins and IP-6

B Vitamins

Cost—Inexpensive
$5 to $10 for 1 to 2 months

Dosage and Type
B-Vitamins—Vegetables, fruits, and beans are good sources of niacin, folic acid, B6, and B12. You may also choose to take them in the form of a general multi-vitamin or multiple B-vitamin.

If you take them in vitamin form make sure you are getting 400 to 800 mcg of folic acid. In addition, make sure that all or most of the other B-vitamins are contained in the supplement, especially B6, B12, and niacin (along with folic acid). If at all possible, make sure you are purchasing niacin, which is better than niacinamide. Niacin has been shown to reduce cholesterol levels, whereas niacinamide has not.

In general, a multivitamin should contain at least 400 mcg of folic acid, 20 mg of niacin, 2 mg of B6, and 6 mcg of B12.

A balanced B-50 or B-complex vitamin will normally contain at least 50 milligrams (50 mg) of the majority of B-vitamins, 50 micrograms (50 mcg) of B12 and biotin (hence the name B-50), and 400 micrograms (400 mcg) of folic acid.

Side Effects
B-vitamins can cause a harmless fluorescent yellow color in the urine.

In general, there are very few side effects associated with B-vitamins when taken in low dosages. It is a good idea to take them with a meal or a short time before or after you eat. Any other side effects associated with B-vitamins usually occur when large doses of one type of B-vitamin are taken.

Niacin can cause an uncomfortable flushing of the skin that feels like a warm sensation and temporarily turns certain areas of your skin red. This generally occurs when your doctor prescribes a large dose of niacin to reduce cholesterol. If this reaction occurs you can take a children's aspirin (81 mg) before you take the niacin or ask your doctor about inositol hexaniacinate, a no-flush niacin.

B-Vitamin Supplements—The Bottom Line
For the Prevention or Recurrence of Prostate Cancer—NO
For Localized Prostate Cancer—NO
For Advanced Prostate Cancer—NO

Please remember that your best source of B-vitamins is from a healthy diet.

IP6
IP6 Supplements—not recommended

IP6—The Bottom Line
For the Prevention or Recurrence of Prostate Cancer—NO
For Localized Prostate Cancer—NO
For Advanced Prostate Cancer—NO

5

Coenzyme Q (CoQ)

In this chapter:

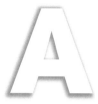

What is Coenzyme Q (CoQ)?

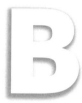

What the Medical Research Tells Us

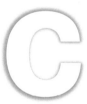

Bottom Line on Coenzyme Q (CoQ)

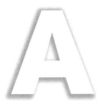

What is Coenzyme Q?

Coenzyme Q is also known as:

CoQ
Coenzyme Q10
CoQ10
Ubiquinone

CoQ is also called ubiquinone because in this case it is ubiquitous, or located in nearly every cell of the human body. CoQ is integral to energy production by various cells of the body, especially the heart cells. Recently, it has received much attention because it also seems to function as a strong antioxidant.

The human body is normally very adept at manufacturing CoQ. The combination of tyrosine (an amino acid found in many foods), vitamins B2, B6, B12, niacinamide, pantothenic acid, folic acid, and vitamin C is used by the body in the creation of CoQ.

In addition, part of the structure of CoQ comes from a substance called mevalonic acid. Mevalonic acid is needed by the liver to produce cholesterol. The enzyme HMG-CoA reductase helps convert a compound in the liver into mevalonic acid, which is later converted into cholesterol. Some cholesterol-lowering drugs work by inhibiting this compound, thereby preventing the manufacture of mevalonic acid—hence lowering cholesterol. Any drug that prevents the manufacture of mevalonic acid also restricts the manufacture of CoQ.

Grocery List

CoQ rich foods:

meat
chicken
(especially chicken hearts)
spinach
sardines
nuts
soybeans

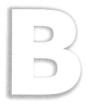

What the Medical Research Tells Us

CoQ and Heart Disease

Most of the research on CoQ has focused on its use for treatment of heart disease, especially congestive heart failure, as well as, high blood pressure, angina (chest and arm pain from heart disease), cardiomyopathy, and mitral valve prolapse.

CoQ and Cancer

Several laboratory studies have shown that CoQ may be helpful for cancer patients who are undergoing chemotherapy. In fact, these studies suggest that CoQ be taken while undergoing any type of chemotherapeutic treatment that might also be toxic to the heart. Keep in mind that there is very limited data currently available. Please talk to your doctor if you wish to take CoQ for side effects caused by a chemotherapeutic drug.

Out of several thousand studies done with CoQ, only about 50 have actually focused on cancer. At this time I prefer to remain cautious regarding its use. There are, however, many cancer patients who take CoQ on a regular basis. Why?

To begin with, a few studies have shown that cancer patients seem to have a lower level of CoQ in their blood. It is very important for you to understand that a reduced level of a particular substance in a cancer patient's blood does not mean that the level should be increased. Secondly, several studies between 1994 and 1995 showed that women with breast cancer were either cured or had partial remission while they took 90 to 390 mg of CoQ a day along with conventional treatment. A closer look is needed.

A number of other studies have indicated that CoQ is not effective. One randomized placebo-controlled clinical trial showed that men who received 90 mg of CoQ a day did not experience a protective effect from oxidative DNA damage when compared to the control group. In fact, the control group (those taking the placebo) had a better result!

This same study also emphasized the past 200+ studies, which have shown a protective effect against cancer by consuming a diet high in fruits and vegetables.

CoQ and Prostate Cancer

There have only been two studies to date on the effect of CoQ and prostate cancer. The first is from the University of Michigan. A hormone-sensitive prostate cancer cell line was used to determine the effect of CoQ. The results were similar to the laboratory studies on breast cancer cells. The more CoQ added to the tumor, the more the tumor grew! It behaved entirely different than expected.

Another small study was conducted with 14 prostate cancer patients who took 600 mg per day of CoQ. In this study the PSA and prostate size decreased for up to one year in ten of the patients. The other four patients did not respond, although each of them had more advanced cancer. The study left many questions unanswered, such as: Did all ten of the men who responded to the CoQ have localized cancer? Were they also receiving conventional treatment?

A final note before we move on: We learned in section A of this chapter that CoQ is composed of many things, including B-vitamins. We also know from Chapter 4 (B-vitamins) that cancer patients should not take excessive amounts of vitamin B supplements, as this can potentially increase the growth of your cancer. Use extreme caution if you are taking CoQ for your cancer and monitor research results.

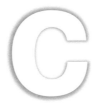

Bottom Line on CoQ

Cost—Expensive

$30 to $100 per month

Depending on the supplement manufacturer there can be a tremendous range in cost. However, they are all expensive. Sixty 100-mg tablets will cost from $30 to $50 per month.

Dosage and Type—Data not complete

Limited studies have tested dosages of from 90 to 600 mg. This wide range and limited number of studies makes it difficult to determine if CoQ is safe and/or effective at this time for the treatment of prostate cancer.

Side Effects

CoQ, much like vitamin K, can interfere with prescribed blood thinners, and cholesterol-reducing drugs can lower blood CoQ levels.

In a recent medical journal it was reported that a 72-year-old woman who was taking a prescription anticoagulant had a reduced response to the drug while taking supplemental CoQ. CoQ is similar chemically to vitamin K. (Vitamin K aids in the process of blood clotting.) If you take a prescription anticoagulant (Warfarin) you need to be sure not to take supplemental CoQ or you may experience reduced effectiveness of the anticoagulant. Talk to your Doctor. Many cancer patients take prescription anticoagulants to thin their blood. Please be careful: These blood thinners are vital for a positive response to therapy and are used to reduce the chance of significant side effects of treatment. For example, estrogen drugs for prostate cancer treatment can cause a serious blockage of blood vessels. This can be prevented if an anticoagulant is prescribed.

Food for Thought

An expenditure of between $30 and $50 per month will cost you anywhere from $360 to $600 per year for CoQ. You would be much better off at this point to use the money instead to purchase fresh fruits and vegetables or plan a special weekend with someone you love.

CoQ—The Bottom Line

For the Prevention or Recurrence of Prostate Cancer—NO
For Localized Prostate Cancer—NO
For Advanced Prostate Cancer—NO

6

DHEA, DHEAS 7-KETO DHEA & Melatonin

In this chapter:

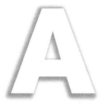

What are DHEA, DHEAS, 7-KETO DHEA & Melatonin?

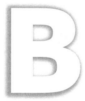

What the Medical Research Tells Us

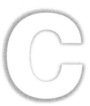

Bottom Line on DHEA, DHEAS, 7-KETO DHEA & Melatonin

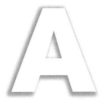

What are DHEA, DHEAS, 7-Keto DHEA, and Melatonin?

DHEA and DHEAs

Dehydroepiandosterone (commonly known as DHEA) is not a vitamin, mineral, or herb. What is it? DHEA is a hormone manufactured by humans and a small number of primates, such as monkeys and apes. Hormones are compounds normally secreted in the blood in very tiny amounts. These hormones travel to other parts of the body to cause an action or actions. For example, the hormone testosterone, largely manufactured in testicles, travels throughout the body and causes multiple effects, ranging from a deeper voice, to hair growth or loss, to determining the sex of a baby. Hormones like testosterone have local effects (e.g., assistance with proper sperm function) and distant effects (e.g., influencing the release of other hormones in the brain). Health professionals and consumers alike need to be careful of the use of hormones, since they are involved in so many bodily functions. While they may help in one situation, they may make another worse, and visa versa.

DHEAS is the same compound as DHEA with a sulfate (S) attached. Both DHEA and DHEAS are manufactured in the adrenal glands, located on top of the kidneys. Smaller amounts are manufactured by the brain, gonads, and skin. The DHEA present in the liver and kidneys also creates DHEAS. DHEAS is by far the most abundant hormone in the human body.

DHEA can be converted to DHEAS, and DHEAS can be converted to DHEA. DHEAS is found in more abundance in the body than DHEA. In fact, blood levels of DHEAS are 300 to 500 times higher than that of DHEA and about 20 times higher than that of any other hormone. More than 99% of the DHEA in the blood is actually in the form of DHEAS. DHEAS attaches itself to a protein as it travels through the blood, which causes it to remain in the bloodstream for an extended period of time. It has a half-life of 10 hours—in other words, it takes 10 hours for 50% of the DHEAS to be used or eliminated from the body. After 20 hours 25% of the hormone remains in the blood.

DHEA, on the other hand, travels unattached through the blood (it has a half-life of 25 minutes). Despite being made in relatively small amounts it is more active than DHEAS when it binds to hormone receptors at different points in the body.

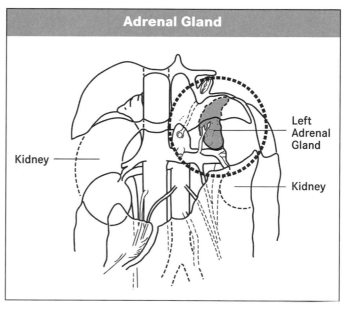

Both DHEA and DHEAS are considered weak androgens or, simply put, they are not as powerful as other hormones. DHEAS is more stable and constant in the bloodstream. If you have your DHEAS level measured you will probably get an accurate reading of the actual amount in your blood. Some DHEA can be converted to DHEAS but with little effect on the actual blood level of DHEAS. However, your level of DHEA can change dramatically during the day (this is called diurnal variation) or from day to day. Both of these hormones travel throughout the body, where they perform many, many tasks, such as manufacturing testosterone, DHT (dihydrotestosterone, a more powerful form of testosterone) and/or estrogen in both men and women.

What causes the release of DHEA and DHEAS? They are controlled by a hormone (ACTH) in the brain that travels to the adrenal glands and signals them to manufacture both. DHEA and DHEAS levels are high in a fetus and low in children, but increase after puberty. They reach their peak at the age of 25 to 30, then slowly decrease with age. In fact, by the age of 70 to 80 there is about an 80 to 90% decrease in the level of these hormones. Men have much more DHEAS (about 10 to 30% more) than women until they pass the age of 50. Once past 50, their level of DHEAS decreases to almost equal that of women. It has been estimated that after the ages of 25 to 30, the level of DHEA(S) decreases in the body at the rate of about 2% a year. Heredity also plays a role in the amount of DHEA(S) in the body. There is a good chance that your body will produce the same amounts of DHEA(S) as either your mother's or father's body.

While many claims have been made, no benefits for DHEA(S) have been proven in significant randomized, placebo-controlled clinical trials. The FDA has not approved the use of this hormone by physicians for any condition, and in fact

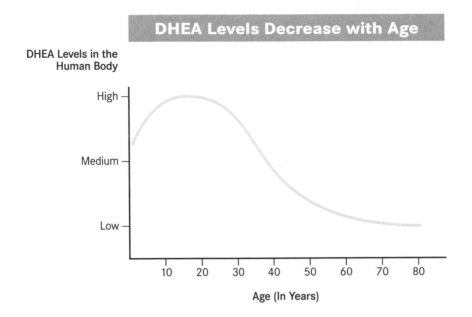

DHEA Levels Decrease with Age

DHEA Levels in the Human Body

banned the sale of DHEA in 1985. The ban was lifted in 1994 with the passage of the Dietary Supplement Health and Education Act. (The Dietary Supplement Health and Education Act places the burden on the FDA to prove that a nutritional supplement is harmful. If a supplement is found to be harmful the FDA can then regulate sales. As a result, many powerful drugs and nutrients—both those potentially beneficial and harmful—are marketed as nutritional or dietary supplements without any proof of safety or effectiveness. The only qualifier required is that the label includes the phrase "no drug intent" and does not claim to help a specific disease or condition.)

A dietary supplement includes any product that contains a dietary substance used to supplement the diet by increasing the total dietary intake of that substance. Sound confusing? It's not, really. Simply put, a dietary supplement such as vitamin B is taken to increase the amount of vitamin B in the body. DHEA is considered a dietary supplement because it is used to increase the amount of DHEA already in the body.

There are no known natural sources of DHEA other than from human or monkey adrenal glands.

7-Keto DHEA

The largest problem with DHEA is the potential for it to produce more testosterone in men and more estrogen in women. Help may be on the way. Henry Lardy at the University of Wisconsin has developed a DHEA called "7-Keto DHEA" which is apparently not converted into testosterone or estrogen. This compound has been shown in animal models not to increase hormone levels, but at the same time it is more potent than regular DHEA. Clinical trials are needed prior to a specific recommendation.

Melatonin

Melatonin, a hormone, is manufactured in the pineal gland, which rests in the center of the brain. Melatonin is key in functions such as puberty, reproduction, sleep cycles, moods, cancer growth, and aging. The formation of melatonin is stimulated by darkness and inhibited by ordinary light. If you draw blood from someone who is sleeping a high level of melatonin will be found, while the opposite is true during the day. Flight attendants who fly all night crossing time zones, elderly people, and individuals who have trouble sleeping tend to have low melatonin levels.

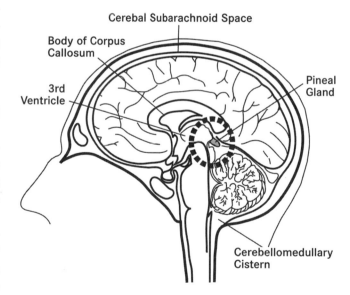

Researchers have found that melatonin can:

► decrease levels of the hormone LH (luteinizing hormone) in the brain. LH travels to the testicles to stimulate the production of testosterone.

► serve as a strong antioxidant in the body. One study found melatonin to be more effective than other antioxidants, such as vitamin E, in protecting DNA and other components of the body from oxidative damage. (These antioxidant properties are normally found when melatonin levels are high as a result of melatonin supplements and not from the levels generated by the pineal gland.)

► potentially boost the immune system. In fact, certain cells in the immune system have receptors for melatonin in order to enhance their function. A number of

79

animal studies have shown that melatonin may also be involved in enhancing other areas of the immune system.

What happens to your sleep pattern if you take supplemental melatonin? Several clinical studies have shown that individuals who take even small amounts of supplemental melatonin (5 mg) are able to increase both sleep and dream time. Other studies have shown that much lower levels (0.1 to 1 mg) may do the same. In fact, 1 to 2 mg, taken for at least 3 to 4 weeks seems to increase the quantity and quality of sleep for insomniacs. Another clinical study observed international flight crew members who took 5 mg of melatonin at bedtime on the day of their return home and for five days afterwards. Researchers found that jet lag, sleep problems, and daytime fatigue decreased among those who took the melatonin and not the placebo. Optimum dosage and use are still being carefully studied.

What the Medical Research Tells Us

A decrease in the levels of DHEA and DHEAS has been associated with increasing rates of disease and even death. Abnormally low or high DHEA levels (depending on the disease and gender) are also found in individuals with chronic diseases and/or the following conditions:

acne
AIDS and HIV infection
Alzheimer's disease and/or dementia
cancer (including prostate cancer)
diabetes
depression
heart disease and other cardiovascular problems, ie., hypertension (high blood
    pressure)

immune deficiency
lupus and other autoimmune conditions, such as rheumatoid arthritis
multiple sclerosis
obesity
work-related stress

Okay, if abnormally low levels of DHEA are found in patients with various diseases, why not just increase the intake of DHEA? Unfortunately, it's not quite that simple. Just because something occurs either before or simultaneously with a disease does not mean that it is responsible for the disease.

It is possible that DHEA can prevent certain diseases and/or indicates disease and/or aging. At this time we are not sure. What we do know is that DHEA has been shown in the laboratory to inhibit chemically induced cancer of the lungs, colon, and skin, and to inhibit spontaneous breast cancer in rodents. However, the problem with many of the animal studies on DHEA is that many of the animals do not manufacture or use DHEA and others produce little. For example, guinea pigs, dogs, pigs, and cattle manufacture little to no DHEA, while mice and rats have levels at least five times lower than humans and primates such as the gorilla and chimpanzee. Other primates, like the rhesus monkey, have DHEA, but still their levels are not equal to that of humans. To observe an effect in these animals, they must be given large quantities of this hormone.

Until recently, researchers were optimistic about the use of this hormone. Several animal studies have now shown that DHEA has caused cancer cells to grow. It is possible that DHEA may increase the risk of cancer in humans and encourage tumor growth.

There have been only a small number of clinical tests done with humans. It is very important to wait and see what additional research indicates regarding the use of DHEA prior to its use for treatment or prevention of disease.

DHEA and Prostate Cancer

What role, if any, does DHEA play in prostate cancer? In both test tube and animal models, DHEA has been shown to have no effect on prostate cancer cells. In one study, DHEA levels were found to be significantly lower among patients with prostate cancer. However, studies of high DHEA levels in prostate cancer patients does not correlate with an increased risk of this disease.

Recently, the *Journal of Urology* reported on a 68-year-old patient with hormone refractory prostate cancer who took DHEA in incremental doses over a period of time. He began with 100 mg twice daily, within four months increased his dosage to 400 mg daily and finally to 700 mg daily. Many of his anemia-related symptoms improved with the use of DHEA. However, facial numbness, pain, and rising PSA (Prostate-Specific Antigen secreted by cells of the prostate gland) and testosterone levels also occurred. DHEA was discontinued six months after its inception. The PSA and testosterone levels decreased, as did the size and hardness of his prostate. At approximately the same time the DHEA was discontinued, diethylstilbestrol (DES—an estrogen) was given to the patient in an effort to cause his refractory cancer to respond to treatment. While this treatment was helpful, it is not known if the response was due to the prior use of DHEA.

Another interesting study was published in May of 1998. Ten cancer-free men of an average age of 60 took approximately 50 mg daily of a DHEA supplement. Researchers found that these patients had a significant increase in DHEA levels, yet their testosterone and PSA levels did not change (compared to the patients who took the placebo). The researchers concluded that "chronic administration of DHEA does not cause a demonstrable affect on testicular function, or on PSA..."

What conclusion can we draw from this? Based on current research, it appears that men who neither have nor are at risk of prostate cancer may be able to take DHEA.

A final comment on the use of DHEA. In a recently published *Journal of the American Medical Association* article it was found that of 16 different commercial DHEA products tested, only 7 contained the actual amount of DHEA advertised on the label. One product contained none, two others had only minimal amounts, and another exceeded the amount advertised on its label. Please make certain you research any product prior to purchase.

7-Keto DHEA

7-Keto DHEA has yet to be tested in prostate cancer patients. If you are interested in this treatment, please talk to your doctor first. And, keep in mind that although the laboratory research is promising, it still needs to be clinically tested with prostate cancer patients.

Melatonin

A recent report from the *Journal of the National Cancer Institute* stated that clinically depressed individuals are more likely to be diagnosed with cancer. Interestingly, lower levels of melatonin have been found in individuals with clinical depression.

Several animal studies have shown that melatonin can inhibit the growth of some cancers. If you restrict melatonin, or remove the pineal gland, the tumors are uninhibited. The vast majority of laboratory studies have shown that a high level of melatonin provides a protective effect against cancer. In fact, lower blood levels of melatonin have been found in some women with estrogen-receptor positive breast cancer. In the laboratory breast cancer cells have been inhibited after melatonin was added to the tumor.

Melatonin may:

inhibit tumor growth
change receptors on the tumor
boost the immune system
behave as an antioxidant

Most of the clinical studies done with melatonin have involved advanced cancer patients. In these studies, melatonin was given in large amounts (20 or more mg per day) in combination with radiation or chemotherapy. In a study of 30 patients with a specific brain tumor, the 16 patients who took melatonin combined with radiation treatment lived longer than the 14 patients who received only radiation. These same researchers did another study with a chemotherapy drug and melatonin supplements for women with metastatic breast cancer. The results were a slower progression of the cancer than normal. It is theorized that the combination of specific chemotherapy drugs and/or radiation with melatonin supplements may increase the effectiveness of treatment. Keep in mind that these studies have been limited in number and relatively small.

Melatonin and Prostate Cancer

In 1987 and 1992, two separate studies found that men with prostate cancer had lower levels of melatonin. Additionally, a 1997 Italian study of prostate cancer patients on LHRH treatment for advanced disease had interesting results. In the study, 14 hormone-refractory prostate cancer patients who were no longer responsive to an LHRH agonist took 20 mg of melatonin per day (in the evening) seven days prior to their LHRH injection. Eight of the fourteen (57%) had a 50% decrease in their PSA. A greater than one year survival rate was seen in nine of the fourteen patients (64%). In addition, three out of five patients with blood platelet problems experienced normal platelet counts. Blood levels of IGF-1 (a possible marker of the severity of the cancer) significantly decreased on this therapy. This preliminary study may indicate that some patients who are hormone-refractory may once again become sensitive to LHRH agonists if they are also given melatonin. A word of caution: this was only one study, and the LHRH agonist used is not available in the United States.

Future use of melatonin for LHRH therapy patients who become hormone-refractory is promising. Melatonin may also provide other benefits. It may help cancer patients who are losing weight with their appetite and may make patients feel better overall. One major side effect of melatonin is that some patients claim it knocks them out or makes them feel sleepy throughout the day.

Much more research is needed, but for now melatonin looks interesting for the treatment of prostate cancer.

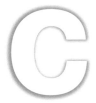

Bottom line on DHEA, DHEAS 7-KETO DHEA and Melatonin

DHEA & DHEAS
Price—Inexpensive
Approximately $5 to $15 per month.

Dosage and Type
Not recommended for treatment or prevention of prostate cancer.

Side Effects
Increased production of testosterone or estrogen. Acne, oily skin, hair growth in women, mood changes, deeper voice. It can potentially increase the risk of or exacerbate prostate cancer.

DHEA and DHEAs—The Bottom Line
For Prevention or Recurrence of Prostate Cancer—NO
For Localized Prostate Cancer—NO
For Advanced Prostate Cancer—NO

DHEA/DHEAS should not be used right now for the following reasons:
▶ We know that DHEA/DHEAS are converted to testosterone.
▶ We know from case studies that it can increase tumor growth.
▶ We know that with the limited amount of data available regarding DHEA/DHEAS and prostate cancer it is safer to place emphasis on the drawbacks rather than positives until more studies are complete.

7-Keto DHEA
Cost—Moderate
The suggested retail price is close to $50 for 60 25-mg capsules.

Dosage and Type
This information is not available presently. Please talk to your doctor if you are considering this treatment.

Side Effects
This is a new supplement—please see your doctor to discuss side effects.

7-Keto DHEA—The Bottom Line
For the Prevention or Recurrence of Prostate Cancer—NO
For Localized Prostate Cancer—NO
For Advanced Prostate Cancer—NO

Melatonin
Cost—Inexpensive
$5 to $10 per month.

Dosage and Type
When at all possible get a good night's sleep. This will allow your body to naturally manufacture melatonin. If you are on hormonal treatment for prostate cancer you may wish to discuss the use of supplemental melatonin with your doctor. Recommended dosage is unknown. If this causes side effects reduce the amount or discontinue use.

Side Effects

May decrease your sex drive and fertility, or cause drowsiness, headaches, depression, and increased allergies. Pay attention to any changes and discuss them with your doctor.

Melatonin—The Bottom Line

For the Prevention or Recurrence of Prostate Cancer—NO
For Localized Prostate Cancer—NO
For Advanced Prostate Cancer—MAYBE

7

Fat, Fatty Acids & Fiber

In this chapter:

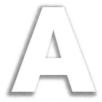

What are Fats, Fatty Acids & Fiber?

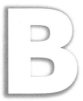

What the Medical Research Tells Us

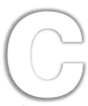

Bottom Line on Fats, Fatty Acids & Fiber

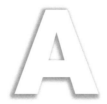

What are Fats, Fatty Acids, and Fiber?

Cholesterol

Cholesterol levels and prostate cancer are somewhat linked. Cholesterol is included in this chapter so that you fully understand how your body responds to fat.

While cholesterol is commonly associated with fat intake it is not always a bad thing. It is manufactured primarily in the liver, with smaller amounts made in the intestines, adrenal glands, and reproductive areas (testicles and ovaries). It is needed to build up cell membranes, and create steroid hormones (testosterone, estrogen), bile acids, (which are needed to eliminate excess cholesterol from the body), and vitamin D. Like fat, cholesterol can add calories and clog arteries.

There are two main classifications of cholesterol; HDL and LDL. HDL, or high density lipoprotein, is the "good" cholesterol. It carries excess cholesterol from different body tissues to the liver, where it is metabolized and processed through the intestines and eliminated from the body. HDL levels can be raised through regular exercise.

LDL, or low density lipoprotein, is the unhealthy cholesterol. It can result in clogged arteries, high blood pressure, stroke, or heart disease. LDL levels can usually be reduced through proper diet.

Fat

What is fat? Fat is a group of compounds composed of one or more fatty acids and glycerol, a compound present in fat. When fats from food are digested in the body, they are broken down into different components. The body changes these components so that they can be carried through the blood.

Fatty tissue or adipose tissue—

These are medical terms for body fat. Energy is normally stored in body fat. It also serves as protection for several organs and can insulate the body from different temperatures. An excessive amount of body fat is harmful. It has been linked to various diseases, such as heart disease, cancer, high blood pressure, and type II diabetes.

Dietary fat

This is the fat found in various foods. Fat from the diet helps provide energy and essential fatty acids. (Some fatty acids cannot be made in the body. They can only be obtained from the diet, and are essential especially for children.) It also carries vitamins A, D, E, and K.

1 gram of fat—9 calories
1 gram of alcohol—7 calories
1 gram of sugar (carbohydrate)—4 calories
1 gram of protein—4 calories

Triglycerides

Triglycerides, composed of three fatty acids, are a major component of the storage of fat in the body. Most of the fat in food is in the form of triglycerides. It has been found that individuals with a higher level of triglycerides are at an increased risk of heart disease. These compounds are measured in the blood.

Fatty Acids

Fatty acids are the building blocks of fat. They are composed of chains of carbon, hydrogen, and oxygen. They differ from one another in two ways: the length of the chain and whether they are saturated or not. Keep in mind that most fats are a mixture of the three major types of fatty acids:

saturated
monounsaturated
polyunsaturated

Saturated fat or fatty acids

Saturated fat contains the maximum number of hydrogen molecules on its chain, hence the title "saturated." Saturated fats, if eaten over a long period of time, can increase your risk of heart disease.

Common sources of saturated fats:
► animal fat, especially from beef
► cheeses made from whole milk or cream

> ► butter
> ► palm oil
> ► coconut oil

Hydrogenated fat or fatty acids

Hydrogenation is the process of adding hydrogen to an unsaturated fat to create a solid saturated fat. If you see a product in the grocery store that says it contains "hydrogenated fat," this is another name for a saturated fatty acid product. (For example, Crisco contains hydrogenated fat.)

Common sources of hydrogenated fat:
> ► Crisco
> ► nondairy creamers
> ► whipped toppings

Monounsaturated fat or fatty acids

One pair of hydrogen atoms on the chain is missing in a monounsaturated fat. (This where the "mono" comes from in monounsaturated.) It is not as compact as a saturated fat and is considered a little healthier.

Common sources of monounsaturated fat:
> ► nuts
> ► pork
> ► oatmeal
> ► canola oil
> ► olive oil
> ► peanut oil

Polyunsaturated fat or fatty acids

In a polyunsaturated fat at least two pairs of hydrogen atoms are missing from the chain. Polyunsaturated fats may reduce blood lipids, but an excess may also lower the protective cholesterol (HDL) as well. There are also a number of specialized polyunsaturated fatty acids, such as omega-3, omega-6, and trans fatty acids.

Common sources of polyunsaturated fat:
> ► soybeans
> ► squash
> ► sweet potatoes
> ► fish

► most vegetable oils: sesame, corn, soybean, and safflower

Omega-3 Fatty Acids

This is a special type of polyunsaturated fat. For example, linolenic acid (an essential fatty acid available only through diet), is a common omega-3 fatty acid. Other sources include cold-water fish, seafood, and fish oil supplements. Flaxseed and flaxseed oil are one of largest sources of omega-3 fatty acids.

Omega-6 Fatty Acids

This is another special type of polyunsaturated fat. Linoleic acid (the other essential fatty acid that can only come from the diet), is a common omega-6 fatty acid. It is thought to influence cardiovascular and growth function when balanced with omega-3 fatty acids. Supplements such as evening primrose, borage, or black currant oil are also good sources of omega-6 fatty acids.

Trans Fatty Acids

These are another special type of polyunsaturated fat. They do not occur naturally in plants and only a small amount is found in animals. Trans fatty acids are processed, and have been hydrogenated to make the fat or vegetable oil more solid. Margarine is a good example. Studies have shown that these fats can raise cholesterol levels in the blood.

Please keep in mind that most oils contain a mixture of fatty acids. Fatty acids, regardless of where they come from, are the building blocks of fat. Often people think that certain oils are very healthy, such as olive oil. Use caution! One tablespoon of olive oil contains approximately 14 grams of total fat (mostly monounsaturated), two of which are saturated fat grams.

Reading Labels

Here is a quick guide to understanding the key words used on food labels:

When the Label Says	It Means
Low Fat	3 grams or less of fat
Less Fat or Reduced Fat	At least 25% less fat
Fat-free	Less than 0.5 grams of fat
Reduced or Less Saturated Fat	At least 25% less saturated fat
Saturated Fat-free	Less than 0.5 grams of saturated fat, and trans fatty acids make up 1% or less of the total fat
Lean	Less than 10 grams of fat, 4.5 grams or less of

saturated fat, and 95 milligrams of cholesterol

Extra Lean . . . . .Less than 5 grams of fat, 2 grams of saturated fat, and 95 mg of cholesterol

Light or Lite . . . . One-third less calories, or 50% less fat

Cholesterol Free . . . . Less than 2 mg of cholesterol and 2 grams or less of saturated fat

Low Cholesterol . . . . 20 mg or less of cholesterol per serving and 2 grams or less of saturated fat

Reduced Cholesterol . . . . At least 25% less cholesterol and 2 grams or less of unsaturated fat

The following words are generally associated with high fat:
au gratin
cream sauce, or creamed
rich
breaded
hollandaise or bernaise
fried, batter-fried, pan-fried

Look for low fat words like:
steamed
au jus
roasted
broiled
poached
stir-fried
grilled

Fiber

Dietary fiber is composed of carbohydrates or complex sugars that are usually not digestible. In other words, it passes through your body and takes a great deal of the "extra baggage" with it. Flaxseed, pectin, cellulose, and lignin contain lots of fiber. Though fiber does not provide any real energy, it does provide a few very big benefits for your health.

▶ Fiber can absorb 10 to 15 times its own weight in water, thereby bringing fluid to the intestines and increasing the movement of the bowels.
▶ Fiber binds to toxic compounds and carcinogens and eliminates them from the body.

► Fiber can lower cholesterol and decrease your risk of diverticulosis and some cancers. However, fiber can also bind to minerals such as zinc and vitamins A, D, E, and K, preventing them from being absorbed by the body. Too many fiber supplements may not be a good idea; however, natural fiber obtained from fruits, vegetables, legumes (beans and peas), whole-grain cereals, and breads is a very healthy plan.

Common Sources of Fiber

Fruit	Fiber (grams)
apple (one)	3.5
pear (1/2 of one)	3.0
prunes (three)	3.0
raisins (1/4 cup)	3.0
raspberries (1/2 cup)	3.0
strawberries (1 cup)	3.0
banana (one)	2.5
orange (one)	2.5
peach (one)	2.0
grapefruit (1/2 of one)	1.5
cantaloupe (1/4 of a melon)	1.0
cherries (five)	0.5

Legumes	Fiber (grams)
baked beans (1/2 cup)	9.0
kidney beans (1/2 cup cooked)	7.5
navy beans (1/2 cup cooked)	6.0
lima beans (1/2 cup cooked)	4.5
peas (1/2 cup cooked)	4.5
lentils (1/2 cup cooked)	3.5

Nuts	Fiber (grams)
peanuts (5 nuts)	0.7
almonds (5 nuts)	0.5

Fresh Vegetables	Fiber (grams)
bean sprouts (1/2 cup)	1.5
mushrooms (1/2 cup)	1.5
tomato (one)	.5
celery (1/2 cup)	1.5
lettuce (1 cup)	1.5
spinach (1 cup)	1.5
cucumber (1/2 cup)	0.5
green peppers (1/2 cup)	0.5

Cooked Vegetables	Fiber (grams)
parsnips (1 cup)	5.5
broccoli (1 cup)	4.5
brussels sprouts (1 cup)	4.5
carrots (1 cup)	4.5
spinach (1 cup)	4.0
sweet potato (one)	3.5
zucchini (1 cup)	3.5
corn (1/2 cup)	3.0
green beans (1 cup)	3.0
kale (1 cup)	3.0
red cabbage (1 cup)	3.0
potato with skin (one)	2.5
asparagus (1 cup)	2.0
cauliflower (1 cup)	2.0
potato without skin (one)	1.5

Breads, Pasta, & Rice	Fiber (grams)
whole wheat spaghetti (1/2 cup cooked)	4.0
bran muffin (one)	2.5
whole wheat bread (one slice)	1.5
brown rice (1/2 cup cooked)	1.0
spaghetti (1/2 cup cooked)	1.0
white bread (one slice)	0.5
white rice (1/2 cup cooked)	0.2

Breakfast Cereals	Fiber (grams)
All-Bran (1/3 cup)	8.5
Bran Chex (2/3 cup)	4.5
Raisin Bran (2/3 cup)	4.0
Shredded Wheat (2/3 cup)	2.5
Grape-Nuts (1/4 cup)	1.5
oatmeal (3/4 cup)	1.5
Cornflakes (1-1/4 cup)	0.5

Keep in mind that the skin from fruits such as apples, peaches, and pears increases the amount of fiber you consume.

A recent study has shown that a high intake of dietary fiber may be linked to a reduced risk of colon cancer. More information is needed to determine if this is factual. At this time it is best for your overall health to consume foods that contain fiber.

What the Medical Research Tells Us

The Diet and Fat Research Controversy

Many dietary studies are retrospective—that is, they seek information about past habits. In the case of diet and fat research, questions are typically asked about what was eaten during the last 5, 10, or even 15 years. These studies are influenced by "recall bias," or the fact that it is difficult to remember diet and supplements from years ago. Think about it. If someone asked you what you had for dinner last Wednesday, could you respond quickly?

Not all dietary studies are retrospective. Prospective studies follow a daily course from the onset of the study into the future. Participants record their dietary intake as they proceed through the trial and report into a clinic periodically. The problem with prospective studies is that if the data are incorrectly reported it affects the results of the study.

Many factors influence the results of any clinical study. For instance, a dietary study done with Eskimos or in the Mediterranean will show that both populations consume a lot of fat. However, their fat intake is significantly different of that of a person from the United States.

Consider also that healthy behaviors tend to breed other healthy behaviors. If a person is cautious about fat intake it is likely that other healthy behaviors are also present.

The message is simple! Studies show that eating more fruits and vegetables and less fat reduces your risk of prostate cancer.

A final point that should be noted about fat studies is that they have gone through quite a bit of change lately. Older studies looked at overall fat consumption, or in other words, how much total fat was consumed in the diet. However, we have learned that the type of fat consumed is crucial in determining your health. It makes a huge difference whether the fat you consume is saturated, monounsaturated, or polyunsaturated. Eskimos eat as much, if not more fat than the average American, but the kind of fat they consume is different. Most of their fat intake is from fish. The omega-3 fatty acids in the fish may be providing benefits beyond knowledge currently available. Researchers have now determined that saturated fat intake may increase your cancer risk (breast, colon, and prostate).

Fat and Prostate Cancer

Please think about your responses to the following rhetorical questions as you read through this portion of the chapter.

▶ Why is it that countries that consume less fat per person tend to have less prostate cancer?

▶ Why is it that autopsy studies on men from different countries, races, and ages show about the same amount of clinically insignificant prostate cancer in men? In other words, prostate cancer occurs just as often in Japanese men as it does in Americans, but our prostate cancers seem to be more clinically significant or dangerous.

▶ Why is it that when a man from another country with a low prostate cancer risk moves to the United States within one to two generations the risk for his family is the same as it is for U.S. men?

▶ Why is the rate of prostate cancer going up in countries that are becoming more similar to the United States?

► Why is it that men who eat diets high in fiber and low in fat seem to have a decreased risk of prostate cancer?

There are many possible answers to these questions. Certainly, increased consumption of fat is one of the answers. Overall behavior habits are another. Common sense dictates that a high intake of fat is unhealthy while a diet rich in fresh fruits and vegetables has been proven to provide numerous health benefits.

Studies done on prostate cancer and fat have shown an increased risk of prostate cancer with a high fat intake.

Laboratory studies have shown that fat can promote the growth of prostate tumors. In an experiment at Memorial Sloan-Kettering, human prostate tumors were grown in animals until they could be felt. Some of these animals were put on a low-fat diet, while others were placed on a high-fat diet. It was found that the animals on the reduced-fat diet (with about 20% of their calories coming from fat) experienced an inhibition of their tumors. Those on the high-fat diet did not see any improvement in the tumors. Additionally, the animals on the reduced-fat diet had lower PSA levels. It is important to note that both diets contained the same number of calories. A final interesting point is that the animals who were placed on *extremely* low-fat diets (less than 20% to as low as 2%) did no better than the animals on *average* low-fat diets (about 20% of their calories from fat). When considering a reduction in the amount of fat in your diet please remember that you do not need to eliminate it completely. Fat is absolutely necessary for energy and for other vital functions.

A generally agreed upon healthy amount of fat in your diet is 20% of your daily intake, with as little as possible from saturated fat—less than 10% of total daily fat intake.

How does fat intake increase the risk of prostate cancer?

Animals that are given testosterone over a long period of time experience growth of prostate tumors. It is believed that fat stimulates the release of testosterone. In both Caucasian and African-American men who reduced their daily fat intake from 40% to 30%, the levels of testosterone and other hormones also decreased.

Low-fat foods may also contain other potentially protective components. For example, fruits and vegetables contain numerous antioxidants, fiber, and other compounds that can potentially inhibit the growth of prostate tumors in the laboratory. A low-fat diet is a win-win situation. First, you are not eating an excessive amount of foods that promote tumor growth, and second, you are consuming foods (fruits and vegetables) with other anticancer compounds.

A recent study in Canada showed that men who consumed high levels of saturated fat were also more likely to be diagnosed with *advanced* prostate cancer. Based on information from this study, it is likely that not only does fat intake increase the risk of prostate cancer, it affects the progression and behavior of the cancer as well.
    A study done in Hawaii found a significant correlation between fat intake and the chance of dying from prostate cancer after the age of 70. Another study also found the same for men in their late 60s to 70s. In both studies the results were the same: a reduction in fat intake had a positive effect on prostate cancer. It appears that men from around the world all have about the same chance of being diagnosed with clinically insignificant prostate cancer as they age. However, several countries known for high fat consumption have more instances of clinically significant prostate cancer.

Fatty Acids and Prostate Cancer

Research on fatty acids is a new territory in the field of prostate cancer. Laboratory studies and animal studies have shown that omega-6 polyunsaturated fatty acids (linoleic acid) can promote the growth of human prostate cancers, whereas omega-3 fatty acids can inhibit their growth. However, there is much controversy surrounding these findings. Please continue to monitor future research results in this area of study. In the meantime, the following charts provide important information on foods that contain omega-3 fatty acids.

Fish	Fat (grams / 100 grams fish)	Omega-3 Fatty Acids (grams / 100 grams of fish)
mackerel	13.9	2.5
herring	9–13.9	1.6
salmon	10.4	1.4
bluefish	6.5	1.4
sardines (in oil)	15.5	1.4
swordfish	2.1	1.4
European sole	1.2	1.3
striped bass	2.3	0.8
rainbow trout	3.4	0.5
tuna	2.5	0.5
halibut	2.3	0.4

Atlantic cod	0.7	0.3
ocean perch	1.6	0.2

Fish Oils	Fat (grams/100 grams of oil)	Omega-3 Fatty Acids (grams/100 grams of oil)
Promega	100	44.2
MaxEPA	100	29.4
cod liver oil	100	18.5

Studies have also shown that eating fish just once or twice a week can significantly reduce your chances of dying suddenly from heart problems. In addition, fish may contain other compounds (such as vitamin D) that are beneficial for you.

The Mediterranean diet, which that has recently been claimed to provide health benefits, is high in omega-3 fatty acids such as olive oil and canola oil. The following vegetable oils also contain omega-3 fatty acids.

Vegetable Oils Omega-3 Fatty Acid Content (grams/100 grams of Oil)	
flaxseed (linseed)	53.3
canola	11.1
walnut	10.4
wheat germ	6.9
soybean	6.8
olive	1.5
corn	1.0
cottonseed	0.5

How do omega-3 fatty acids work? They may be converted in the bloodstream into a substance that reduces inflammatory conditions in the body, thereby inhibiting cancer growth. On the other hand, omega-6 fatty acids may be converted into a substance that does just the opposite, thereby promoting the growth of cancer.

However, much more work needs to be done to determine exactly what role omega-6 fatty acids play in overall health. Studies have shown that some omega-6 fatty acids may be good for you. *The American Journal of Clinical Nutrition* recently published a review of all the papers done on linoleic acid (an omega-6 fatty acid). Authors P.L. Zock and M.B. Katan stated, "Although current evidence cannot exclude a small increase in risk, it seems unlikely that a high intake of linoleic acid substantially raises the risks of breast, colorectal, or prostate cancer in humans."

Fiber (including Pectin and Modified Citrus Pectin) and Prostate Cancer
Laboratory, animal, and several human studies have shown that dietary fiber can lower your risk of prostate cancer and/or prostate cancer progression. Studies on modified citrus pectin (by Kenneth Pienta, M.D., University of Michigan, co-author of *The ABC's of Advanced Prostate Cancer*) in animals have shown that it can slow progression of prostate cancer and prevent tumors from attaching to various components of the blood and thereby spreading throughout the body. In these animals it prevented metastasis but did not slow growth of existing tumors. However, until additional clinical studies are completed citrus pectin is not recommended as a substitute for natural fiber.

Once again, data on dietary fiber found in fruits and vegetables indicates this is the better route for good health. In a study with vegetarians who consumed fiber from natural sources it was discovered they had lower levels of testosterone than non-vegetarians. This seems to indicate that dietary fiber may work by lowering levels of certain hormones (e.g., testosterone) in the body that promote prostate cancer growth and progression. Regardless, a diet complete with natural fiber increases your chance of good health and may reduce your risk of prostate cancer.

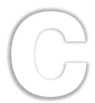

Bottom Line on Fat, Fatty Acids, and Fiber

Cost—Inexpensive
The price of regular fruits and vegetables is very reasonable—far less than the cost of supplements.

Dosage & Type
In this case, more is better. Eating a variety of fruits and vegetables will keep you interested and provide your body with numerous healthy compounds.

Side Effects

The fiber in some foods and over-the-counter fiber products may provide too much "laxative effect" or bowel problems. If this happens, reduce the dosage or amount of fruits and vegetables you eat.

Fat, Fatty Acids, and Fiber—The Bottom Line

For the Prevention or Recurrence of Localized or Advanced Prostate Cancer—YES

About 20% or less of your total daily calories should come from fat—especially saturated fat, which should be no more than 10% of your total daily fat intake. Replace your milk with soy milk and/or use skim milk. Increase your natural dietary fiber intake. Maintain a normal cholesterol level. The omega-3 fatty acids in canned tuna (packed in water) are good for you in moderation. Substitute olive oil or canola oil for your current cooking oil, although remember to use any oil in moderation.

8

Flaxseed & Soy

In this chapter:

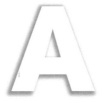

What are Flaxseed & Soy?

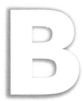

What the Medical Research Tells Us

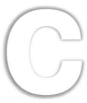

Bottom Line on Flaxseed and Soy

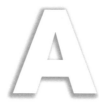

What are Flaxseed and Soy?

Flaxseed

"Phytoestrogen" is a term used in cancer research today. What does it mean? Phytoestrogen is just a fancy term for foods or plants that contain a natural source of estrogen. Soy, the most popular phytoestrogen currently, contains natural plant estrogens that are also referred to as "isoflavonoids" or "isoflavones." However, another fabulous source of phytoestrogens is flaxseed. Flaxseed is a tiny seed that is used to make linseed oil and is the largest source of "lignans," another class of phytoestrogens. Lignans are also found in a variety of other foods, such as lentils and garlic, although the largest source is flaxseed.

What's the rage about phytoestrogens? Countries that consume a large amount of phytoestrogens typically have low rates of cancer—particularly prostate and breast cancer.

Flaxseed is available in a variety of forms at your local health food store or supermarket:

  plain flaxseed
  flaxseed meal
  flaxseed flour (or powder)
  flaxseed capsules
  flaxseed oil

Lately flaxseed oil and capsules have received much attention. Books, magazines, and health professionals are touting them as a sort of cure-all, for everything from allergies to cancer. Use extreme caution with both the oil and the capsules, as they contain a high amount of fat. In fact, if you look at a flaxseed oil label you will see that it contains a number of calories—almost all of which come from fat! (Chapter 7, on Fat, Fatty Acid, and Fiber, explains the dangers of a high intake of fat in regard to prostate cancer.) Additionally, flaxseed capsules and oil are quite expensive. Flaxseed oil is thick, tastes horrible, and needs to be refrigerated. Despite all the press, it is not a very good source of plant estrogens. When the oil is taken out of flaxseed, many of the plant estrogens are lost. And, regardless of what is advertised, such as the new high-lignan flaxseed oils, you still need 4 to 6 tablespoons of the oil to equal the same amount of plant estrogens in just 1 tablespoon of flaxseed. You may wish to spatter a little in salads or on pasta, but try not to heat, cook, or bake flaxseed oil.

For the following reasons—including to avoid the fat—I recommend that you just buy plain old flaxseed (just the seeds):

► It's inexpensive. (For a dollar you can buy a month's supply.)
► It has a lower quantity of fat than flaxseed oil and capsules.
► It is a good source of omega-3 fatty acids (the beneficial fatty acids found in fish like tuna and salmon).
► It is a good large source of fiber (which has been linked to lowering your chances of getting cancer and heart disease).
► It is a large source of plant estrogens or lignans.
► It contains protein, calcium, potassium, B-vitamins, iron, and boron (which may be essential for bone health).

There are two easy ways to eat flaxseed. First, you can simply swallow 1 to 2 teaspoons of plain flaxseed daily. In other words, just put them in your mouth and drink a little water or soda and they go down quite easily. Second, you can grind up the seeds with a coffee grinder and add the powder to your juice. Flaxseed powder contains most of the active ingredients in flaxseeds. However, after grinding the seeds you need to ingest the powder within 10 to 20 minutes or it will oxidize and may lose its effectiveness. Flaxseed meal and flour are good also; they are just a little more expensive than flaxseed. You can add flaxseed to almost any soup, sauce, salad, yogurt, or juice.

Minerals/Vitamins in Flaxseed	
Minerals (per gram of flaxseed)	Amount
iron	175–225 mcg
zinc	100–150 mcg
manganese	50–70 mcg
copper	20 mcg
potassium	10 to 14 mg
phosphorus	8 to 12 mg
magnesium	6 mg
calcium	4 to 5 mg
sulfur	4 mg
sodium	0.5 mg

Vitamins (IU or mg per 100 grams of flaxseed	
vitamin A	19 IU
niacin (vitamin B3)	9 mg
vitamin B	60.8 mg
vitamin E	0.6 IU
vitamin B1	(thiamine)0.5 mg
vitamin B12	(cobalamin)0.5 mg
vitamin B	20.2 mg

Flaxseed also contains:

► high amounts of insoluble fiber and some soluble fiber, which can lower cholesterol levels, keep you regular, and change your hormone levels in a more favorable way (lower testosterone, for example). Pectin is an example of a fiber that works in the same way.

► 18 of the 20 amino acids (which are the building blocks of proteins) found in nature. It contains low levels of methionine, an amino acid. High levels of methionine have been discovered to promote tumor growth in the laboratory.

► high protein.

► high levels of healthy fatty acids, mostly in the form of alpha-linolenic acid (omega-3 fatty acid), which can be converted into healthy antiinflammatory and disease preventing compounds.

Soy

As of late, soy has become an extremely popular product. As we discussed earlier in this chapter, soy contains phytoestrogens. The soybean is the source of so many different soy products that it has become almost impossible to keep up with them. The following list contains the most popular soy products. There are hundreds of soy products currently available on the market.

Young Soybeans/"Edamame"

Edamame is steamed over boiling, salted water until heated thoroughly. It is considered a Japanese specialty and sold in pods, shelled, canned, or frozen. It is an excellent source of B-vitamins (Folic acid), fiber, calcium, and unsaturated fat.

Miso and Miso Soup

Miso is a thick aged paste, made from soybeans, salt, and a fermenting agent (usually a mold culture). At times a grain, like rice or barley, is added for extra flavor. Miso soup is a common appetizer and breakfast drink in Japan. It has a strong flavor. It is high in sodium and low in protein, but it is also a good source of plant estrogens and many enzymes that are helpful for digestion. There are three basic types of miso:

► Hacho—made of only soybeans. Aged in wooden kegs for up to three years. It is the strongest of the three.

► Kome—made of soybeans and rice. Aged for six months. It is the mildest form of miso.

▶ Mugi—made of soybeans and barley and has a milky look. It is aged for approximately 18 months.

Natto—Fermented and Cooked Soybeans

Natto is used in Japan as a spread or in soups. It is high in protein and fiber and lower in sodium than either miso or soy sauce. It contains iron, other minerals, and B-vitamins. However, since it is a fermented soy product with tyramine (an amino acid), it may raise one's blood pressure if one is taking an antidepressant MAO inhibitor.

Okara

Okara is the pulp remaining after soy milk is strained. It is a good source of protein and fiber, and may help lower cholesterol. It is used in granola, cookies, and vegetarian burgers. It needs to be refrigerated and used within a few days.

Soybeans

Soybeans are the bean from which most soy products are made. In their natural state, soybeans are the best source of plant estrogens. They can be either boiled or steamed. A half of a cup of soybeans has the same amount of protein as an 8-ounce glass of milk. They are also a good source of vitamin C, iron, calcium, and folic acid. If you have trouble digesting soybeans, try using Beano, a product available in health food stores that will help prevent digestive problems sometimes caused by soybeans.

Soybean Lecithin

Soybean lecithin is made from soybean oil. It is an emulsifying compound used in bakery foods, candy products, and chocolate coatings, as well as in nonfood products, such as cosmetics, rubber, plastics, paints and inks, etc. Choline is derived from lecithin in the digestive tract and carried to the brain, where it is made into a compound that is involved in memory. The brain does not manufacture choline on its own.

Soybean Sprouts/Young Soybean Plants

These are sometimes difficult to locate. Ask your health food shopkeeper to order them for you. Soybean sprouts are tasty, low in sodium, and filled with nutrients.

Soy Cheese

Soy cheese is formed with vegetable gums and contains a milk-derived product called "calcium caseinate," or isolated soy protein, which is dairy-free. It is low in calories and fat. Soy cheese is also lactose and cholesterol-free.

Soy Flour/Ground Whole Dry Soybeans or Defatted Soybean Flakes

Soy flour is a simple form of soy protein with very little starch. It contains a large amount of protein and improves baked goods. Store it in the refrigerator or freezer for maximum freshness.

Soy Grits

Soy grits taste like soybeans but they cook faster. They are good for thickening chili, stews, and spaghetti sauces. Try soy grits as a substitute for ground beef or add it to your ground or chopped meats to cut the fat.

Soy Milk

Soy milk is used as a base for tofu, soy yogurt, and soy cheese. It is one of the most popular soy products on the market because it can be easily substituted for your regular milk. It's available in plain, vanilla, chocolate, strawberry, and carob flavors, it's sold in low-fat and no-fat types, and even comes in small 8-ounce sizes. Soy milk is lactose-free, so it is easily digested. (However, it should not be used as a substitute for infant feeding formulas.) It contains about the same amount of protein as cow's milk, without the hormones (like BGH, bovine growth hormone) and cholesterol, has one-third the fat of milk, and has fewer calories and more B-vitamins. Try to use a soy milk fortified with calcium, vitamin D, beta-carotene, and other B-vitamins. You can drink soy milk straight, or use it in baked goods, cereal, or in any recipe that calls for milk. You can store unopened soy milk for up to one year. Once opened, refrigerate and use within five to seven days.

Soy Nuts

Crunchy, delicious soy nuts can be easily eaten anywhere. The are an excellent source of potassium. You can make your own soy nuts by soaking dried soybeans overnight in the refrigerator, then draining and spreading on an oiled baking sheet. Season with a little tamari (soy sauce), garlic powder, cayenne pepper, or cinnamon, and then roast at 350 degrees Fahrenheit for one hour, or until golden brown. For a healthy treat, add soy nuts to the next batch of cookies or brownies you bake.

Soy Oil

Soy oil is used in a large number of vegetable oils, mayonnaise, margarine, salad dressings, salad oils, vegetable shortening, coffee whiteners, creamers, sandwich spreads, liquid shortening, and supplements. Soy oil does not have the same health benefits of most other soy products, although it does contain a high omega-3 fatty acid content.

Soy Protein Powder

Soy protein powder is similar to soy flour except that the soybeans are first cooked and then ground while the soy flour is dried (not cooked) and ground. The powder is finer than the flour and has less of a bean taste. It can be used in soy milk, for baking, and in various drinks.

Soy Sauce

Soy sauce contains little to no plant estrogens. Many commercial brands are also filled with sugar, caramel coloring, and MSG, a food additive that has been linked to allergic reactions, headaches, and heart palpitations. Furthermore, it normally contains high levels of sodium and tyramine, which are known to raise blood pressure. In Japan soy sauce is still aged in wooden kegs by several manufacturers. There are two basic types of soy sauce:

> ► Shoyu (sometimes known as tamari shoyu) is usually allowed to ferment slowly for a little more than one year. It is made from defatted soybean meal, wheat, water, and sea salt. Shoyu is used in cooking and as a condiment. It has a sweet flavor.
> ► Tamari is a wheat-free shoyu with a stronger and deeper flavor. It has a higher content of glutamic acid (a more natural and gentler version of MSG). Tamari is used in soups or as a marinade.

Soy Supplements

Soy supplements (also known as soy isoflavones) are a fairly new product. Please talk to your doctor prior to using soy supplements. They are a concentrated source of plant estrogens that may increase your estrogen level. Very little research has been completed on this product, so it is important to approach it with caution. Also, keep in mind that natural soy products, like soybeans, have a variety of healthy compounds in them that might not be contained in the supplement.

Soy Yogurt

Soy yogurt is lactose- and cholesterol-free. Pretty tasty, too!

Tempeh

Tempeh is a great source of plant estrogens. Tempeh is processed much the same as blue cheese. It has a firm, springy texture and a rich, mushroomy flavor that ranges from smoky to nutty. It is often used for grilling and stir-frying, and is substituted for beef in soups, chili, and casseroles. If you may notice specks of gray or black in the tempeh, don't panic—this is because it is naturally fermented. Tempeh will keep in the refrigerator for about seven days and in the freezer for up to six months. The fermentation of the soybean improves the protein and B-vitamin content and removes the gas-producing bacteria so you experience little or no flatulence. Tempeh is high in fiber and omega-3 fatty acids. Try it baked, broiled, grilled, stir fried, as a pizza topper, in salad, etc.

Textured Vegetable Protein

Also known as texturized soy protein, this soy product is often used instead of hamburger to make vegetarian chili, sloppy joes, tacos, meatballs, and veggie burgers. Textured vegetable protein makes the most of vegetarian meals. It is isolated soy protein without the carbohydrates. Textured vegetable protein (TVP) has a meaty texture, but without the cholesterol and calories of meat. To use TVP, first rehydrate it (almost a full cup of boiling water for 1 cup granules or chunks). Let it sit for 5 minutes, add to your recipe and simmer another 15 to 20 minutes. Stored in an airtight container in a cool, dry place, it will remain fresh for several months.

Tofu

Tofu (also known as bean curd) is sometimes called "meat without bones" or "meat of the fields" because of its high protein and mineral content. Lui An, a Chinese ruler, is believed to have created Tofu in 200 B.C. It is believed that Buddhist monks took the soybeans from China to Japan sometime during the sixth to eighth centuries. In the twelfth century, monks opened vegetarian restaurants in their temples and the Japanese public sampled their first tofu. However, it was not until the 1980s that tofu became more common in American markets. Tofu is sold in many different forms:

> ► Firm tofu (or extra-firm)—Pressed so there is less moisture and a concentration of nutrients. Must be refrigerated.
> ► Regular tofu (or soft)—Soft with delicate texture. Must be refrigerated.
> ► Silken tofu—Sweet with a custard-like texture. It is usually packaged in shelf-stable boxes.
> ► Smoked tofu—Precooked in soy sauce seasoning and then smoked, this

tofu has a soft brown color and a nice flavor. It has a firm cheese-like texture. Should be refrigerated.

▶ Dried tofu—This is freeze-dried, stored at room temperature, and boiled in water. It has a more chewy and flexible texture and can be eaten anywhere.

▶ Tofu pouches (also called "age," which is pronounced "AH-gay")—Deep-fried cubes that are hollow inside. Must be refrigerated or frozen.

▶ Frozen tofu—This can change the texture from soft to more chewy.

Both firm and soft tofu are used for cooking. Silken tofu works best for blending because of its texture. It is fairly easy to locate tofu with a low fat content. Please be careful when buying tofu to check for freshness (look for an expiration date on the package) especially if it is floating in water—it may contain harmful bacteria. The best way to purchase tofu is in a sealed package. Cook at a high temperature until it reaches an internal temperature of 160 degrees Fahrenheit. Fresh vacuum-packed tofu can be kept for three to five weeks in the refrigerator. Pasteurized tofu can be stored longer.

Keep your tofu in the refrigerator at all times—it spoils quickly. If it is purchased in bulk or removed from its sealed package, it should be stored in a covered container submerged in water that is changed daily. Fresh tofu has no odor and a smooth (but not slick) surface. If it smells funny or becomes slippery to the touch then it is probably spoiled—throw it away!

Tofu is high in protein and calcium. Both the firm and extra-firm tofu have more water removed from them, thereby increasing the protein and calcium content. Check the label for the saturated fat content, compare it to others, and choose the best one for your needs. Tofu is like a miniature sponge, making it excellent for soaking up flavor. In warm dishes like soups (it is commonly found at the bottom of a miso soup bowl in Japanese restaurants) and/or sauces it absorbs the flavor of the dish you are eating. Experiment with tofu. Food is a matter of taste: what one person likes another doesn't, and visa versa.

The following chart is from the U.S. Department of Agriculture. Keep in mind that tofu contains no cholesterol, and that although approximately 50% of the calories in tofu come from fat it is not saturated fat. Also, generally the softer the tofu, the lower the fat content.

1/2 Cup of Tofu (4 ounce) Contains:			
	Firm Tofu	Soft Tofu	Silken Tofu
calories	120	86	72
protein (grams)	13	9	9.6
carbohydrates (grams)	3	2	3.2
fat (grams)	6	5	2.4
saturated fat (grams)	1	1	0
cholesterol	0	0	0
sodium (milligrams)	9	8	76
fiber (grams)	1	0	0
calcium (milligrams)	120	130	40
iron (milligrams)	8	7	1
% calories from protein	43	39	53
% calories from carbohydrates	10	9	17
% calories from fat	45	52	30

Yuba

Yuba is the skin from hot soybean milk obtained during processing. It is commonly consumed in China and Japan. It is often used in these countries to make imitation meat. Fresh yuba can be shaped and served cold, fried, or in a broth. This meatless product is sold under such names as "Molded Pig's Head" and "Buddha's Duck." It has a high protein content and can be used in stews and soups.

Other Soy Products

The list is gigantic. As time marches on we may find soy in nearly everything. Included is a list of a few of the many other soy products available:

▶ soy "meats"—soy burgers and soy hot dogs ("Bocca Burger," "Smart Dogs," "Gimmie Lean," "Italian Links")
▶ tofu cream cheese
▶ tofu dips
▶ tofu ice cream
▶ tofu mayonnaise
▶ tofu ravioli

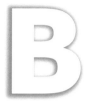

What the Medical Research Tells Us

Flaxseed

The lignans in flaxseed are metabolized in the body into enterodiol and entero-lactone, two protective steroids. The following chart indicates the amount of lignans contained in some popular foods. Please note that flaxseed, lentil beans, triticale, and soybeans are excellent sources of plant estrogens, along with a host of vegetables and fruits.

Source of Lignan (g)	Total Lignans (mcg)	Enterodiol (mcg)	Enterolactone (mcg)
flaxseed	500-700	80-90	580-600
lentil beans	17-18	7-8	10
triticale (cereal)	9-10	5-6	4
soybeans	8-9	6-7	1-2
oat bran	6-7	2-3	3-4
wheat bran	5-6	2-3	3
kidney beans	5-6	3-4	2-3
wheat (cereal)	4-5	4-5	0-1
navy beans	4-5	3-4	1-2
garlic	4-5	0-1	3-4
sunflower seeds	4	2	2
asparagus	3-4	1-2	2-3
carrots	3-4	2-3	0-1
oats (cereal)	3-4	2-3	0-1
brown rice	3	1-2	1-2
sweet potatoes	3	2-3	0-1
corn (cereal)	2-3	2	0-1
broccoli	2-3	1-2	0-1
pinto beans	2	1-2	0-1

pears	1-2	1-2	0-1
rice bran (cereal)	1-2	1-2	0-1
rye (cereal)	1-2	0-1	0-1
plums	1-2	0-1	1
barley (cereal)	1-2	0-1	0-1

The largest source of lignans are plain, inexpensive flaxseed. One clinical trial showed that the quantity of lignans in the body increased with the consumption of carrots, spinach, broccoli, and cauliflower. Men showed higher increases than women, suggesting a possible gender difference in intestinal metabolism of lignans.

Flaxseed and Cancer

The reality of the situation is that flaxseed has undergone very few studies when it comes to disease, especially cancer. However, the early data on flaxseed indicates that it may be extremely beneficial in the fight against cancer, so we should see a number of new clinical trials in a very short time.

The urinary excretion of lignans (an indicator of lignan amount in the body—the higher the excretion rate, the more lignan there must have been in the body) has been shown to be significantly lower in breast cancer patients and individuals at high risk of breast and colon cancer compared with that of vegetarians. Lignans have also been shown to inhibit estrogen-sensitive breast tumors in the laboratory. In addition, flaxseed given to female rats inhibited the onset and progression of breast cancer, and flaxseed given to male rats with chemically induced colon tumors also inhibited disease.

A recent study has shown that giving ground flaxseed to mice prior to implanting melanoma or skin cancer resulted in a significantly reduced metastasis and inhibited the growth of other tumors. In fact, the more flaxseed the mice received, the lower the number of tumors. The authors concluded that, "...flaxseed may be a useful nutritional tool to prevent metastasis in cancer patients."

As a result of preliminary studies it is believed that flaxseeds may possibly bring some benefit by:

► acting as estrogenic agents in some cases
► acting as antiestrogenic agents in other cases
► acting as strong antioxidants
► blocking tumor growth
► blocking the conversion of hormones to other hormones that may stimulate cancer growth
► inhibiting angiogenesis (or the growth of new blood vessels by tumors)

► increasing the amount of sex hormone-binding globulin (also known as SHBG). SHBG can bind to hormones and make them less available to other parts of the body and cancers (therefore, the less the amount of hormone(s) available to the cancer, the less fuel it has to grow)

► acting as immune system enhancers

► being a good source of omega-3 fatty acids, mostly alpha-linolenic acid, which has been found in numerous studies to possibly reduce the risk of cancer

More good news regarding these studies! There were very few to no side effects observed in the animals taking flaxseed. Keep in mind also that flaxseed and soy are both strong sources of plant estrogen. It is likely that since soy has been found to be potentially beneficial in the area of prostate cancer flaxseed may see similar results.

Soy

Is soy really as good as it sounds? Natural soy products contain many different healthy compounds, in addition to the plant estrogens. Let's take a look at some of the other beneficial compounds found in the soybean or soy products:

boron
B-vitamins
calcium
coenzyme Q
fiber
inositol hexaphosphate (IP6)
iron
isoflavones
lecithin
magnesium
omega-3 fatty acids
phytates and phytic acid
phytosterols
polyphenols
protease inhibitors
protein (and amino acids)
saponins
terpenes
vitamin E
low methionine concentration*

*Methionine is one of 20 amino acids that are needed to make proteins. It has to be obtained from the diet because the body cannot make it from another source. This makes methionine an essential amino acid. Soybeans contain 10 of these amino acids. They are:

Amino Acid in Soy	Amount
leucine	7.6
lysine	6.6
isoleucine	5.8
valine	5.2
phenylalanine	4.8
threonine	3.9
tyrosine	3.2
cystine	1.2
tryptophan	1.2
methionine	1.1

Methionine is found in the smallest quantity of all the amino acids in soybeans. Why is this important? Several studies have looked at soy's ability to reduce tumors in rats. In these studies the effects of soy were reversed when greater quantities of methionine were added to the diet. In addition, when the rats were initially given casein (a protein found in cow's milk) and later switched to soy the tumors were inhibited. What might all this mean? The amount of the essential amino acid methionine in soybeans is less than that found in cow's milk. The lack of methionine in soy products may be one of the many reasons that soy inhibits tumor growth in the laboratory.

The Specific Plant Estrogens or Isoflavones in Soy

The topic drawing the most attention regarding soy is the plant estrogen, or isoflavones, it contains. Isoflavones are the most common type of phytoestrogens. The two major isoflavones in soy are genistein and daidzein. Isoflavones are found in many different plants, including fruits and vegetables, and especially leguminous plants, and contain a large concentration of soy. Different soy products have different quantities of plant estrogen. For example, soybeans, tofu, tempeh, and soy protein are good sources, whereas processed soy products like soy hot dogs, hamburgers, and tofu yogurt may only have about 10% of the isoflavone content of other products.

So, with this in mind let's take a look at the total isoflavone content, including the genistein content (the most potent isoflavone in soy) of some popular soy products.

Soy Product	Total Isoflavones (mcg/gram)	Genistein (mcg/gram)
soybeans	1,200-4,200	650-2,700
roasted soybeans	2,700	1,425
soy flour	2,000	1,450
textured vegetable protein (TVP)	2,275	1,180
soy protein powder	625-1000	375-650
tempeh	870	420
tofu	300-530	185-250
miso	390-650	225-280
tempeh burger	385	260
tofu yogurt	280	160
soy hot dog	240	130
soy cheese	45-20	05-60
soy milk	30-90	20-60
soy sauce	0	0

Soy Product	1 Serving	Isoflavones
soybean	1/2 cup	175-200
tempeh	4 ounce	60 mg
soy protein powder	1/3 cup	45 mg
tofu	4 ounce	40 mg
soy milk	1 cup	20 mg
soy sauce	–	0

Soybeans (or roasted soybeans) are usually the largest source of plant estrogen, while soy protein powder and tempeh contain a moderate amount, soy milk contains a small amount, and soy sauce is worthless in terms of plant estrogen content. The more you manipulate the soybean, the more likely it is that you lose plant estrogen.

In Asian countries soy is most often served in the form of miso, soymilk, tempeh, or tofu.

Soy and Prostate Cancer

The prostate cancer death rate in Asian countries is very low compared to that of the United States. For example, prostate cancer death rates are somewhere between four to seven times lower in Japan than in the United States. The number of prostate cancer incidences among both Japanese and American men seems to be even, but American men have more clinically significant prostate cancer, which leads to a higher fatality rate. A recent table published in the *Journal of the National Cancer Institute* (90:21: 1637-1647, Nov. 4, 1998) shows the death rate from prostate cancer in various countries and the average life expectancy of men from each country:

Grocery List

Sources of Plant Estrogens:

apples
barley
cherries
coffee
garlic
green beans
licorice
oats
parsley
pomegranates
potatoes
red clover
rice
wheat
yeast

Country	Prostate Cancer Deaths	Average Life Expectancy
New Zealand	35 men out of every 100,000	73
Belgium	34 men out of every 100,000	73
United States	32 men out of every 100,000	75
Austria	31 men out of every 100,000	74
France	31 men out of every 100,000	75
Australia	30 men out of every 100,000	74

Canada	29 men out of every 100,000	73
England	28 men out of every 100,000	74
Italy	23 men out of every 100,000	74
Greece	16 men out of every 100,000	74
Singapore	7 men out of every 100,000	72
Japan	6 men out of every 100,000	77
Hong Kong	5 men out of every 100,000	75

These figures indicate that while the life expectancy is nearly equal the prostate cancer fatality rates are significantly different. What is the reason for this? New Zealand has a higher fatality rate from prostate cancer than the United States. However, they also consume more meat and less fish than Americans. What about Italians and Greeks? They consume less meat and much more fiber and they have a much lower death rate from prostate cancer. How about men living in Singapore, Japan, and Hong Kong? They eat much less meat and much more fish, fiber, and soy products.

Studies have shown that men in Asian countries consume on the average of about 50 to 100 mg of isoflavones (soy) daily compared to approximately 1 to 5 mg per day for American men.

If we could delay the clinically significant prostate cancers by several years the prostate cancer death rates would be greatly affected. Why? In approximately 25% of the new cases of prostate cancer the patient is less than 65 years old. Most of the benefits of soy for treatment of prostate cancer have been conducted in the laboratory, although several human studies have also been interesting. Genistein has been shown to inhibit both hormone-sensitive and hormone-insensitive cells in the laboratory. It has also been shown to reduce the metastatis of prostate cancer in the laboratory. In a human study, isoflavones seem to be much more concentrated in the prostate than in the blood. A case study published in the *Medical Journal of Australia* reported on a 66-year-old man who consumed 160 mg of plant estrogen (from red clover) daily for one week before a radical prostatectomy (complete removal of the prostate). Upon analysis after the surgery it was found that the prostate had both mild and strong areas of cancer cell degeneration, but no changes were seen in the normal prostate cells. This pattern looked similar to men on hormonal ablation or synthetic estrogens for the treatment of prostate cancer.

Laboratory studies have shown that plant estrogens may also prevent prostate cancer by:

► decreasing blood androgen (male hormone) levels

► increasing the concentration of SHBG (sex hormone-binding globulin)—a protein that can bind to male hormones and prevent them from being used by the prostate to stimulate the growth of cancer

► binding to hormone receptors—so that even if a hormone is available it cannot bind to the prostate

► inhibiting 5-alpha reductase—an enzyme in the prostate that converts natural testosterone into a more powerful testosterone called DHT (dihydrotestosterone)

► restricting other enzymes associated with cell growth

► causing direct tumor destruction—such as antiangiogenesis—which does not allow the cancer to make more blood vessels (thus starving the tumor).

► decreasing IGF-1—increased levels of IGF-1 (Insulin Growth Factor) have recently been shown to be a potential marker for increased risk of prostate cancer in several clinical human studies

Soy and Hot Flashes from Prostate Cancer Treatment (Hormonal Ablation)

It has been shown in clinical studies that soy effectively reduces hot flashes in menopausal women. Therefore, the research team at the University of Michigan studied five men experiencing severe hot flashes from hormonal ablation treatment for prostate cancer. All five experienced at least a 50% reduction in the number of hot flashes, along with a decrease in the severity of the hot flashes, within two to four weeks of consuming one serving of soy daily along with 800 IU of vitamin E. One man had such severe hot flashes before the study that he considered discontinuing hormonal ablation because the hot flashes kept him awake most of the night. While only a preliminary study, the results were very encouraging. A much larger study is currently being conducted.

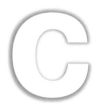

Bottom Line on Flaxseed and Soy

Flaxseed

Cost—Inexpensive
For $1 to $2 you can buy a month's supply of flaxseed.

Dosage and Type
1 to 2 teaspoons or tablespoons of flaxseed daily.

Side Effects
Intestinal discomfort. Some people cannot tolerate seeds. If this is the case, try grinding them into a powder. Prescription medicines should not be taken at the same time of day as flaxseed (the high amount of fiber may not allow the absorbtion of your medication by the body).

Flaxseed—The Bottom Line
For the Prevention or Recurrence of Prostate Cancer—MAYBE
About 1 to 2 teaspoons or tablespoons of flaxseed daily. Do not use flaxseed oil or capsules.

For Localized Prostate Cancer—MAYBE
At least 1 to 2 teaspoons or tablespoons of flaxseed per day. Do not use flaxseed oil or capsules.

For Advanced Prostate Cancer—MAYBE
At least 1 to 2 teaspoons or tablespoons of flaxseed a day. Do not use flaxseed oil or capsules.

For Hot Flashes from Hormonal Ablation Treatment for Prostate Cancer—MAYBE
Approximately 1 to 2 teaspoons or tablespoons of flaxseed daily. However, if you are taking flaxseed for localized or advanced prostate cancer you do

not need to increase the dosage. Do not use flaxseed oil or capsules.

Soy

Cost—Inexpensive

Soy milk runs $1 to $2 per carton. Tofu and/or soy protein powder should only be a few dollars per month.

Dosage and Type

Focus on soybeans, soy protein powder, tofu, and soy milk. They are the easiest to find and contain high levels of plant estrogens.

Side Effects

Gastrointestinal upset. Iron overload (very high doses).

Soy—The Bottom Line*

For the Prevention of Localized or Advanced Prostate Cancer—YES

At least one or more servings (more is better) of soy products daily. Miso, soy milk, soy protein powder, tempeh, soybeans and tofu are among the most highly recommended.

For Hot Flashes from Hormonal Ablation Treatment for Prostate Cancer—YES

At least one or more servings (more is better) of soy products daily. Miso, soy milk, soy protein powder, tempeh, soybeans and tofu are among the most highly recommended.

In addition, you can also take 800 IU of vitamin E in divided daily doses with food (400 IU in the morning, and 400 IU at night). Results take 2 to 4 weeks.

If you have localized or advanced prostate cancer, we are not sure if soy provides any benefit right now. However, getting 1 serving a day may be helpful and has been shown to reduce total cholesterol levels.

9

Garlic & Garlic Supplements

In this chapter:

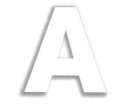

What is Garlic?

What the Medical Research Tells Us

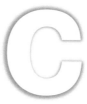

Bottom Line on Garlic

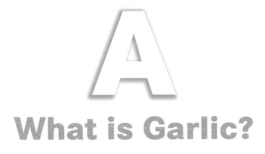

What is Garlic?

Garlic has a very interesting history. It has been used for thousands of years to treat a variety of problems. The Chinese used it to treat high blood pressure, the Europeans used it for bubonic plague, and the Egyptians believed that it could increase physical strength. During a number of wars garlic was placed on wounds as an antiinfection agent. In southern Europe, where individuals consume large quantities of garlic, heart disease is low, and some believe that garlic is partially responsible for the benefits of the Mediterranean diet.

Garlic is one of more than 500 members of the allium plant family. Several other well-known members of the same family include:

chives
onions
shallots
leeks

When raw garlic is cut or crushed, the enzyme allinase combines with a sulfur compound in the garlic to make allicin. Allicin is responsible for the aroma and taste of garlic. However it is not stable and it breaks down in just a few hours at room temperature or after about 15 to 20 minutes of cooking. This instability makes it difficult to study its actual medical effects. Allicin protects garlic against bacteria and other harmful organisms. It is one of the most powerful substances in chopped or crushed garlic.

There has been a virtual avalanche of printed, radio, and television ads regarding the use of garlic supplements. As a result it is one of the most popular over-the-counter products available. Are garlic supplements really good for you?

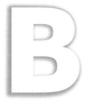

What the Medical Research Tells Us

Garlic, Garlic Supplements, and Cancer

Many studies have shown that among populations that consume high amounts of garlic, onions, leeks, and shallots (all members of the same plant family) there is a lower rate of overall cancer.

A prospective study done in the Netherlands followed a total of 120,852 men and women who took garlic supplements, and ate onions, and leeks for more than three years. It was determined that garlic supplements, and ate onions, and leeks did not reduce the risk of colon cancer in men, nor did it reduce the risk of breast cancer in women. The same group was then analyzed for the risk of lung cancer. Again, the researchers found that onions, leeks, and garlic supplements did not reduce the risk of lung cancer, and many of the participants in the group were nonsmokers.

However, in a population study done among women from Iowa, there was a decreased risk in lung cancer for women who ate a lot of vegetables, including leeks and fresh garlic. This observation was also found in a Chinese study, where many of the individuals also consumed chives, onions, and natural garlic. This evidence would seem to point to the likelihood that fresh onions, leeks, and garlic do provide benefits while supplements do not.

Garlic and Garlic Supplements and Prostate Cancer

A recent study discovered an association between increased consumption of both natural garlic and garlic supplements and a lower risk of prostate cancer. The study found that individuals who consumed natural garlic at least twice a week had a lower risk of prostate cancer. It also determined that individuals who took garlic supplements along with natural garlic also had a lower risk, although not as low as the garlic only group. In conclusion, this study found that men who consumed natural garlic, vitamin B6, beans, or peas on a regular basis had a lower risk of prostate cancer.

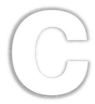

Bottom Line on Garlic and Garlic Supplements

Cost—Very Inexpensive
Natural garlic, onions, leeks, shallots, etc., are available everywhere and at a fraction of the cost of garlic supplements.

Dosage and Type
Do not take supplements—garlic, onions, and leeks in natural form only, please!

Side Effects—Increased Flatulence and Gastrointestinal Upset
Garlic can cause stomach upset and increased amounts of gas. If this happens just reduce the amount of garlic you eat. It may thin your blood also. Talk to your doctor if you are taking a prescribed anticoagulant.

Garlic and Garlic Supplements—The Bottom Line
For the Prevention or Recurrence of Localized or Advanced Prostate Cancer
Garlic—MAYBE Supplements—NO
In natural form, please. Adding natural garlic to your diet several times a week is a wonderful and healthy idea.

10

Lycopene

In this chapter:

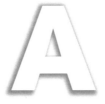

What is Lycopene?

What the Medical Research Tells Us

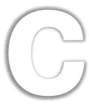

Bottom Line on Lycopene

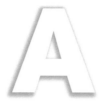

What is Lycopene?

A long time ago the tomato was considered a poisonous fruit to be completely avoided. The truth is, not only is the tomato not dangerous, it is one of the safest and healthiest foods a person can eat! It was brought to Spain from Mexico in the 1500s and worked its way across Europe and eventually became a major influence in Italian food preparation. It was not widely accepted as safe to eat until the 1800s. Today, almost 70 million tons of tomatoes are grown around the world each year, with about 9 million tons of that from the United States. Most of the commercial tomatoes are used in foods such as ketchup, soups, salsas, and sauces. They are a good source of many healthy compounds, including vitamins A, C, E, folic acid, potassium, and other trace elements, such as flavonoids, phytosterols, and lycopene.

Lycopene is just one of the hundreds of carotenoids found in nature. As you may recall from Chapter 3, carotenoids are natural pigments thought to be helpful in the prevention of some diseases, including cancer. It is the carotenoids in tomatoes that makes them red. Most carotenoids, including lycopene, are not converted into vitamin A.

Laboratory studies have proven lycopene to be one of the strongest antioxidants in nature. It is found in very high concentration in tomatoes, tomato products, and several other foods. In fact, more than 80% of the lycopene intake in the United States

Food	Amount of Lycopene (mg per 100-gram Serving)
tomato powder	100-125
dried tomato in oil	50.0
canned pizza sauce	13.0
ketchup	10-13
tomato soup	8.0
tomato sauce	6.0
tomato paste	5.0-150
tomato juice	5.0-12.0
fresh guava	5.0
cooked tomatoes	4.0
guava juice	3.0
raw pink grapefruit	3.0
fresh watermelon	2.0-7.0
fresh papaya	2.0-5.0
fresh tomatoes	1.0-4.0
dried apricot	1.0
canned apricot	0.1
apricot	less than 0.01

comes from tomato products. Other common foods that contain lycopene are listed in the table on the previous page.

Cooked tomatoes contain even more lycopene. The heat releases lycopene from the food's specific storage area and makes it more available to be absorbed by the body.

Lycopene is stored in a few areas of the body. The prostate, testicles, adrenal glands, and liver each contain high levels of lycopene.

A few additional notes on lycopene:
► Sunlight may reduce lycopene levels.
► Other supplements and healthy nutrients probably have little effect on lycopene concentration.
► Smoking and drinking probably have little effect on lycopene levels.
► Cooking releases additional lycopene.

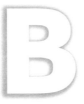

What the Medical Research Tells Us

Lycopene, Tomatoes, and Cancer

A summary of all the past tomato studies was recently published by the Journal of the National Cancer Institute. This analysis looked at 72 past studies on tomato intake and cancer incidence. It was found in 57 of the 72 studies that tomato intake was linked to a reduced risk of cancer. In 35 of the studies this link was statistically significant.

Lycopene may be responsible for a significantly reduced risk of prostate, lung, and stomach cancer.

Products such as raw tomatoes, ketchup, salsa, tomato paste, tomato soup, and spaghetti sauce are not only tasty—they're good for you! In addition, cooking and/or processing tomatoes does not diminish this effect. The author of this analysis, Dr. Edward Giovannuci of Harvard University Medical Center, also stated that lycopene supplements have not been proven or disproven to have the same effect as tomatoes or tomato products at this time.

Lycopene, Tomatoes, and Prostate Cancer

In a study of 14,000 men who ate tomatoes more than five times a week (versus those who ate less than one serving a week), prostate cancer risk was reduced. The largest tomato and prostate cancer study conducted by health professionals showed a 35% decrease in prostate cancer risk among individuals who ate more than ten servings a week of tomato products. It was further determined from this study that the consumption of tomato products also decreased the risk of being diagnosed with advanced or aggressive prostate cancer. Tomato sauce was associated with the lowest prostate cancer risk, with tomatoes and pizza showing a moderate decrease while tomato juice provided little protection.

There is currently very little information available on lycopene supplements and reduced prostate cancer risk. One study (at the Karmanos Cancer Institute in Detroit, MI) looked at men getting lycopene supplements (10mg twice a day) for 3 weeks before having prostate surgery. They seemed to benefit, but these results are too preliminary to make any conclusion right now.

Lycopene Supplements—Antioxidant or Prooxidant?

In Section A of this chapter it was mentioned that lycopene is believed to be one of the strongest antioxidants in nature. Remember, though, that in certain situations antioxidants can also act as prooxidants. Lycopene supplements have not been tested thoroughly at this time, and may in fact act as prooxidants in terms of prostate cancer. A recent study was done on mice with human prostate cancers. One group of mice were given lycopene supplements and the other group of mice were not. It was found that the mice on lycopene supplements had a greater increase in their prostate cancer than the other group of mice. Why? The lycopene supplement may have acted as a prooxidant and encouraged tumor growth.

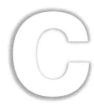

Bottom Line on Lycopene

Cost—Inexpensive

Tomatoes and tomato products are not expensive and there are so many wonderful foods you can prepare with them. Do not use lycopene supplements at this time. It is expected that more data will be published in the future.

Dosage and Type

Eat tomatoes or tomato products several times a week. Review the list of other foods that contain lycopene and make every effort to incorporate a variety of them in your daily diet. Stay away from lycopene supplements for now.

Side Effects

No known side effects.

Lycopene—The Bottom Line

For the Prevention or Recurrence of Prostate Cancer—YES, Supplements—NO
For Localized Prostate Cancer—YES, Supplements—NO
For Advanced Prostate Cancer—YES, Supplements—NO

It has been demonstrated that an increased consumption of tomatoes and tomato products is linked to a decreased risk of prostate cancer and possibly a lower risk of aggressive prostate cancer.

11

PC-SPES

In this chapter:

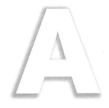

What is PC-SPES?

What the Medical Research Tells Us

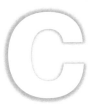

Bottom Line on PC-SPES

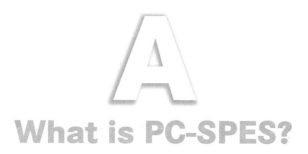

What is PC-SPES?

PC-SPES (the PC stands for "prostate cancer," and spes is the Latin word for "hope") is a combination of eight different herbs that are said to have been used in Chinese medicine to treat cancer. Each 320-mg capsule contains a combination of the following herbs:

Isatis indigotica (da qing ye)
Glycyrrhiza glabra and Glycyrrhiza uralensis (gan cao)—licorice
Panax pseudo-Ginseng (san qi)—ginseng
Ganoderma lucidum (ling zhi)
Scutellaria baicalensis (huang qin)—skull cap
Dendranthema morifolium Tzvel—chrysanthemum
Rabdosia rebescens
Serenoa repens—saw palmetto

PC-SPES has been commercially available since November, 1996. It has recently gained a tremendous amount of attention because it has significantly decreased PSA levels in some prostate cancer patients.

What the Medical Research Tells Us

Each 320 mg capsule of PC-SPES contains a combination of the eight herbs listed in Section A. However, the quantity of each herb is currently unknown. PC-SPES has been advertised as a nonestrogenic food supplement (it contains no estrogen), but several of its components have definite estrogenic activity. For example, in an estrogen binding test licorice combined with estradiol and ginseng has shown estrogen-like potential.

In one of the PC-SPES studies, published in the *New England Journal of Medicine*, researchers found that PC-SPES demonstrated strong estrogenic activity in yeast, mice, and humans. Eight hormone-sensitive patients took PC-SPES for at least one month, during which time a dosage of at least four 320-mg capsules was taken daily for two straight weeks. The PC-SPES significantly decreased the serum testosterone and PSA levels—almost equal to the levels seen with LHRH treatment and estrogen treatment in other studies.

After a period of time, six of the patients discontinued PC-SPES and saw an increase in their PSA within two to six weeks after cessation of treatment. All eight patients experienced erectile dysfunction and breast tenderness, and one patient had superficial venous thrombosis (a blood clot, usually in the leg). These side effects are similar to those previously observed in clinical trials using a synthetic estrogen (or LHRH agonist) for metastatic prostate cancer.

The University of Michigan recently published a paper on the effect of PC-SPES for treatment of localized prostate cancer. One patient had a PSA of 8.8, which decreased to an undetectable level (about zero) after approximately two months on PC-SPES (nine capsules per day). His side effects included severe breast enlargement, erectile dysfunction, a low testosterone level, loss of body hair (especially on the arms and legs) and swelling in his ankles. On the good side, his hairline did not recede any further.

After decreasing his PC-SPES intake to six capsules a day, his PSA level remained undetectable. A few months later he decreased his dosage to five capsules a day and finally to four capsules daily. His PSA remained undetectable throughout the entire time he took PC-SPES. His side effects also remained the same, with the addition of an increase in total cholesterol and a decrease in LDL (the unhealthy cholesterol). These side effects parallel those of men on estrogen treatment.

Why Not Just Use Prescribed Estrogen?

Studies done in the '60s and '70s found that most prostate cancer patients who took a dosage of 5 mg daily of DES (diethystilbestrol—a prescribed estrogen) experienced beneficial results. *(PSA tests were not yet available to determine if a patient had prostate cancer or the effect of treatment on prostate cancer.)* There were, however, a number of cardiovascular problems reported with this dosage.

As a result, researchers decided to test lower doses of DES to determine if the effects on prostate cancer would remain constant while at the same time decreasing cardiovascular side effects. At a dosage of 3 mg the side effects were drastically reduced, and positive results for the prostate cancer were noticeable within one month of initial intake of DES. In some cases a dosage of as little as 1 mg daily of DES was also effective.

The introduction of PSA testing led to an interesting study in 1994. It was discovered that 98% of the men (with various degrees of prostate cancer) who participated in the earlier DES studies had PSA levels of less than 4 ng/mL (nanograms [billionths of a gram] per milliliter) within three months of initial doses of DES. Approximately 50% of the total 98% had undetectable levels of PSA. It is remarkable how well estrogen reduced PSA levels! Other types of low-dose and prescribed estrogen have also shown very good results.

One of the questions most frequently asked by prostate cancer patients is "Why aren't we using estrogen treatment for prostate cancer?" The answer is simple. While the controversy that arose in the '60s and '70s over the dosage of estrogen and its side effects continued, hormonal ablation was introduced as a new treatment. It was discovered that hormonal ablation (a process during which an LHRH agonist is injected into the body) reduces testosterone and PSA levels without the cardiovascular side effects. Doctors in the United States soon prescribed LHRH agonists over estrogen treatment. Once this shift to hormonal ablation began, the use of estrogen treatment faded quickly into the past. In addition, the uses of synthetic estrogen for localized or locally advanced prostate cancer is controversial. Although PSA and primary-tumor volumes decrease, some patients continue to have signs of tumor growth and spreading with treatment at earlier stages of the disease.

PC-SPES Versus Hormonal Ablation or Prescribed Estrogen

There are two primary questions at this time regarding the use of PC-SPES:

► Does PC-SPES provide any additional benefit over hormonal ablation or estrogen treatment?
► Should PC-SPES be combined with conventional treatment to provide additional benefits for patients?

The answers to these questions currently remain a mystery. Clinical trials are yet to be conducted that compare conventional treatment with PC-SPES treatment. The introduction of PC-SPES to the consumer marketplace has caused the renewed debate over low dose prescribed estrogen for the treatment of prostate cancer. Clinical trials are needed.

The parallel effective dosage of DES versus PC-SPES seems to be 3 mg per day, although we are not absolutely certain how many capsules of PC-SPES should be taken. A good starting place seems to be from three to six 320 mg capsules daily, with higher dosages if the cancer is hormone-insensitive.

▶ If you are considering PC-SPES for treatment of prostate cancer, discuss it thoroughly with your doctor.

▶ Record dosage and effect so that you can discuss your particular situation without having to recall specifics from memory.

▶ Remember that side effects are reduced with lower doses.

▶ PC-SPES apparently should be taken on an empty stomach at least two hours before or after a meal because of its reduced effectiveness when combined with food.

Hormone-Insensitive (Hormone-Refractory) Prostate Cancer

Commonly, after a patient stops responding to hormone ablation treatment he is given second line hormonal treatments such as estrogen and/or chemotherapy. This is the one situation in the United States when estrogen is still used for treatment of prostate cancer. Since PC-SPES behaves in much the same manner as estrogen, it is not unlikely that it may develop a significant role for advanced patients. Among patients who are using PC-SPES there have been cases when they no longer responded to prescribed estrogen and/or chemotherapy but had positive results from PC-SPES.

PC-SPES: Putting All the Pieces Together

Physicians and patients need to educate themselves about PC-SPES. This supplement has many possible advantages, disadvantages, and similarities to prescribed estrogen and LHRH treatment.

Similarities Between PC-SPES and Prescribed Estrogen or LHRH Treatment

▶ substantial decrease in testosterone and PSA within two to six weeks

▶ alternative treatment for hormone refractory cancers.

▶ side effects such as breast tenderness, loss of libido, and swelling or clotting in the legs (circulation problems).

▶ possible reduction of cardiovascular risk factor and the need for periodic cholesterol evaluations.

▶ need to be on prescribed anticoagulants to prevent coagulation problems (venous thrombosis) at higher PC-SPES dosages (9 capsules/day).

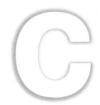

Bottom Line on PC-SPES

Cost—Very Expensive

No insurance reimbursement or coverage available. The approximate cost is $60 for 108 capsules. Three capsules a day equals $162 a month, or $1944 a year. Six capsules a day equals $324 a month, or $3888 a year. Nine capsules a day equals $486 a month, or $5832 a year.

Dosage and Type

One to nine 320-mg capsules a day. A dosage of three to six capsules a day is the most generally preferred treatment. Over time the dosage may be reduced if the PSA level remains stable. PC-SPES at higher dosages (9 capsules/day) should probably be taken with a prescribed anticoagulant. Talk to your doctor before you begin taking PC-SPES!

Side Effects

Breast enlargement or tenderness, erectile dysfunction, loss of sexual drive, swelling, loss of body hair and change in cholesterol level.

PC-SPES—The Bottom Line

For the Prevention or Recurrence of Prostate Cancer—NO
For Localized Prostate Cancer—MAYBE
For Advanced (hormone-insensitive) Prostate Cancer—MAYBE
For men experiencing hot flashes from LHRH treatment (PC-SPES is estrogenic, thus it may reduce hot flashes)—MAYBE

12

Selenium

In this chapter:

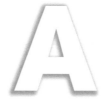

What is Selenium?

What the Medical Research Tells Us

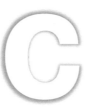

Bottom Line on Selenium

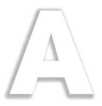

What is Selenium?

Selenium is a "trace mineral" because it is needed only in very small quantities. It is normally sold in micrograms (mcg, or a millionth of a gram). Selenium is a popular antioxidant because it works directly with an enzyme in the body to prevent free radical damage. Additionally, it works closely with vitamin E to prevent damage to the body.

Selenium Levels Found in the Soil in the United States

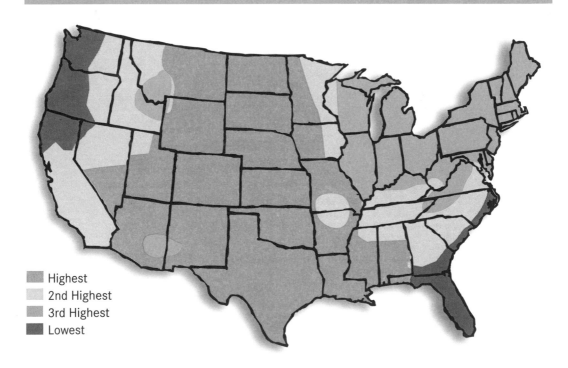

Highest
2nd Highest
3rd Highest
Lowest

Over the past 35 years researchers have noticed that in certain areas of the world where the level of selenium in the soil is low, there is a higher risk of many diseases, including heart disease and cancer. In the United States, where the selenium level in the soil varies from region to region (depending on rainfall), there is a relationship between the selenium level and disease. (The level of selenium in the soil affects the level of selenium found in the foods we eat.) As a general rule, the more rainfall in an area, the less selenium in the soil.

The soil in central areas of the United States contains the highest levels of selenium, while the Northwest Pacific, some eastern states, and Florida contain the least.

Grocery List

Sources of Selenium:

wheat germ	garlic
Brazil nuts	onions
bran	turnips
wheat	rye
oats	soybeans
brown rice	mushrooms
barley	

What the Medical Research Tells Us

Selenium and Cancer

A higher risk of cancer has been linked to a low selenium intake since 1969. In the laboratory, when selenium is added to different cancers it has inhibited their growth.

How does selenium work?

▶ Selenium may function as an antioxidant, increasing the levels of glutathione peroxidase, a substance that assists in blocking free radicals in the body.

▶ Selenium may behave similarly to aspirin, reducing the levels of prostaglandin E2, which in turn may prevent some cancers. (Please refer to Chapter 2—Aspirin.)

▶ Selenium may repair damaged cells or cause abnormal cells to die, thereby slowing the growth of tumors.

Selenium and Prostate Cancer

It has been known for some time that there is a link between selenium intake and prostate cancer. Selenium consumption has been decreasing over a period of time in Britain and parts of Europe, possibly due to a decrease in selenium-rich imported North American flour. Studies have shown that the average current intake of selenium in these areas may be only about 30 to 40 mcg a day. As the selenium intake has declined, the number of prostate cancer incidences has advanced.

The first double-blind, placebo-controlled cancer prevention study to test the effectiveness of selenium was conducted at the University of Arizona. The researchers in this study were initially trying to determine if selenium could reduce the risk of skin cancer recurrence. (All the participants had previously had some type of skin cancer.) Men and women were recruited from seven dermatology clinics located in low-selenium regions of the United States. The candidates took 200 mcg of selenium daily in the form of a 0.5-gram high-selenium brewer's yeast tablet. The average length of time in the study for each participant was 4-1/2 years. The selenium supplement increased their natural level by nearly 70% without any significant side effects. The results of the study were a surprise to everyone. Selenium had no effect on skin cancer. However, there was:

▶ a 37% decrease in overall cancer incidences
▶ a 46% decrease in lung cancer
▶ a 58% decrease in colorectal cancer
▶ a 63% decrease in prostate cancer

Since the publication of this trial in the 1996 *Journal of the American Medical Association*, several other studies have published results that support the theories of the initial trial.

Selenium, Vitamin E, and Cancer

It is possible that selenium and vitamin E may work better together to enhance each other's effect at reducing the risk of prostate cancer. The National Cancer Institute has established a multisite clinical trial to test the combination of selenium and vitamin E on cancer, including prostate cancer. Since both selenium and vitamin E have demonstrated positive results on their own, this study may lead to some very exciting new information.

▶ Low levels of selenium have been associated with a higher risk of some cancers, including prostate cancer.

► A dose of 200 mcg a day of selenium has been associated with a reduction in the number of localized and advanced prostate cancers.

► Dietary intake of selenium-rich foods is linked to a 50 to 75% decrease in advanced prostate cancers.

► A dose of 200 mcg of selenium daily is inexpensive and safe.

► Selenium is difficult to obtain from foods in large quantities. (Brazil nuts contain a good amount, but also contain Barium which may be toxic at high dosages.)

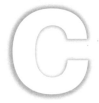

Bottom Line on Selenium

Cost—Inexpensive
Average cost of supplements is approximately $5 to $10 per month.

Dosage and Type—200 mcg a day.
Please look for a brand that includes the word selenomethionine—ideally a yeast-based tablet. This is the same type of selenium supplement that was used in the successful clinical trial. Always take with a meal. The most effective dosage for prostate cancer is from 100 to 200 mcg per day.

Side Effects
Gastrointestinal upset, increased flatulence, and possible hair, tooth, and nail problems.

Always take selenium with a meal. Most of the side effects can be reduced or eliminated if selenium is taken with food. If you experience continued side effects after taking with a meal, try decreasing the dosage slightly.

Selenium Supplements—The Bottom Line
For the Prevention or Recurrence of Prostate Cancer—YES
For Localized Prostate Cancer—MAYBE
For Advanced Prostate Cancer—MAYBE

13
Shark Cartilage

In this chapter:

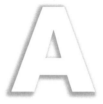

What is Shark Cartilage?

What the Medical Research Tells Us

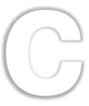

Bottom Line on Shark Cartilage

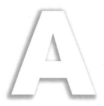

What is Shark Cartilage?

Shark Cartilage

The skeleton of a shark is composed of cartilage, not bone. The popular shark cartilage supplement is made by drying the cartilage, pulverizing it into a powder and then packaging the powder in capsule form. Why all the excitement? A few years ago a national television program proclaimed the benefits of shark cartilage for men in America. The study that this television program was based on only tested 19 patients. The sad truth is that the majority of research and studies do not support this theory.

The theory behind shark cartilage supplements is that they have shown limited potential as an antiangiogenic. Cancerous tumors require blood vessels and nutrients to grow. An antiangiogenic restricts blood vessel growth and therefore the supply of nutrients to a tumor. In the few studies that have been completed to test this theory the shark cartilage itself has been used, not the supplement. Shark cartilage may also contain antiinflammatory properties and the ability to reduce damage caused by free radicals. Overall research is very limited.

Worth Mentioning—Shark Liver Oil and Bovine Cartilage

Both shark liver oil and bovine (cow) cartilage are being advertised as possessing anticancer properties. Neither has adequate research to support their use. A number of cases have been reported in which prostate cancer patients who experienced urinary incontinence as a result of their surgery successfully used bovine cartilage supplements to treat their condition. Please do not begin using either of these products until further research has been conducted.

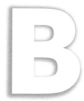

What the Medical Research Tells Us

Shark Cartilage, Cancer, and Prostate Cancer

Various cancers depend on blood supply to continue living, growing, and moving. This is called "angiogenesis," or the growth of new blood vessels. If researchers can prevent these new blood vessels from forming, there is a possibility that cancers can be destroyed. The University of Michigan has done a number of studies in which it has been shown that the more aggressive the cancer the more blood vessel growth is present. Aggressive tumors require nutrients carried by the blood to grow.

There are some components in shark cartilage itself (not necessarily the supplement) that have shown potential antiangiogenic activity. However, these are isolated components of the cartilage that have been concentrated and may be potent in very small quantities. Shark cartilage has been used experimentally to promote wound healing and to treat inflammatory conditions. For example, a study from Canada using a component from shark cartilage called AE-941 was tested on the forearms (topically) of patients with psoriasis (an inflammatory condition that affects the skin). The shark cartilage demonstrated an ability to reduce the inflammation associated with this disease. Other components from shark cartilage have been shown to have other antiinflammatory properties and the ability to reduce some damage by free radicals. Overall, though, the research is still very limited in this area.

More recent studies done by Canadian researchers have shown that a liquid extract taken from shark cartilage has shown limited ability to reduce blood vessel formation. This agent has inhibited the growth of various breast, ovarian, and other cancer cells in the laboratory. It was also able to reduce the growth of lung cancer cells in mice when given along with cisplatin (a common chemotherapy drug used in cancer treatment). This agent is now being tested in a phase I/II clinical trial in the United States and in Canada.

Objective data on the anticancer and antiangiogenic properties of shark cartilage supplements are not currently available.

A small study, in which orally administered powdered shark cartilage was tested on 12 advanced, hormone-refractory patients, was recently presented from William Beaumont Hospital in Royal Oak, Michigan. Patients were given 1 gram per kilogram daily of shark cartilage for 20 weeks and 10 grams daily thereafter for maintenance. The average age of the patient was 73; average PSA was 47 ng/mL at the beginning of the study. Within the first eight weeks six patients had to withdraw from the study because they could not tolerate the shark cartilage. Another patient had to stop taking shark cartilage after 12 weeks because his disease had progressed rapidly. Among the five patients who were able to complete the first 20 weeks, all had an increase in their PSA. It was concluded in this study that powdered shark cartilage was not effective in treating advanced (hormone-refractory) prostate cancer.

Recently, a larger study of patients with various types of cancer was published in the November, 1998 *Journal of Clinical Oncology*. The following 60 adult patients with advanced, previously treated cancer were enrolled in this study:

16 breast cancer patients
16 colorectal cancer patients
14 lung cancer patients
8 prostate cancer patients
3 non-Hodgkins lymphoma patients
1 brain cancer patient
2 unknown primary source cancer patients

Patients were given orally 1 gram per kilogram daily of shark cartilage powder, in three divided doses, taken before meals. The powder (5 grams per teaspoon) was mixed in fruit juice. Ten of the patients refused to continue the study or were not able to be located after six weeks of treatment. Five other patients were taken off the study because of gastrointestinal problems or other side effects from the shark cartilage. In 22 of the patients the disease advanced after 6 to 12 weeks. Five patients died of cancer during the study. Six of the eight prostate cancer patients experienced disease progression within 12 weeks; in two others it took longer than 29 to 46 weeks to see progression of the cancer. There were no overall partial or complete responses to shark cartilage treatment out of all 60 patient studies.

The shark cartilage was found to be ineffective as a single treatment agent and had no beneficial effect on the quality of life of these patients.

Other studies of shark cartilage have been published but have not been peer-reviewed. For example, a noncontrolled study of shark cartilage treatment was published in 1996. Fifteen of the twenty-one patients in the study were treated conventionally with surgery, chemotherapy, or radiation. Shark cartilage was given (1 gram per kilogram daily) to patients who had no signs of disease after the conventional treatment. Researchers claimed a 61% decrease in tumor size, which was they believed was due to the shark cartilage. Quality of life was claimed to have improved in 87% of the patients, but the researchers did not explain how this was determined.

The real excitement with shark cartilage research is not in the present supplements but in potentially identifying a few compounds in shark cartilage that may really have some anticancer effects.

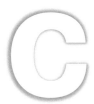

Bottom Line on Shark Cartilage

Cost—Expensive
A few months' supply can cost as much as $50 to $100.

Dosage and Type—N/A

Side Effects
Gastrointestinal upset, nausea, and in rare cases liver problems.

Bottom Line—Shark Cartilage
For the Prevention or Recurrence of Prostate Cancer—NO
For Localized Prostate Cancer—NO
For Advanced Prostate Cancer—NO

Shark cartilage supplements:

full of fillers
very expensive
enormous recommended daily dosage (from the supplement companies)

14

Tea & other Polyphenols

In this chapter:

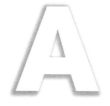

What is Tea?

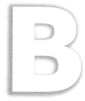

What the Medical Research Tells Us

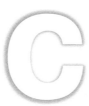

Bottom Line on Tea

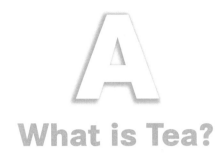

What is Tea?

Green, Oolong, and Black Teas

People all around the world have enjoyed drinking tea for thousands of years. It is possible that in addition to its delicious flavor, tea is also one of the healthiest beverages available and may prevent heart disease and cancer.

Legend has it that tea was discovered in 2700 B.C. when a Chinese emperor sat in the shade of a wild tea plant to relax. A couple of tea leaves fell into his cup of hot water and, voila, tea was discovered. In 800 A.D. a Buddhist monk who was studying in China clipped some seeds from a tea plant and took them home to Japan. By the late 1700s Europeans were widely consuming tea. Today water is the only beverage in the world consumed more than tea.

- ► India is the largest producer of tea—more than 670 million pounds annually.
- ► China grows 600 million pounds of tea per year and exports only 70 million pounds.
- ► Black tea is the #1 tea consumed in the United States and the world.
- ► Green tea is most often consumed in both China and Japan.

The tea plant, which can grow to an average height of 30 feet, is the source for all three types of tea: green, oolong, and black. The only difference between the three types is how they are processed.

- ► Green tea leaves are lightly steamed or dried—unfermented
- ► Oolong tea is partially fermented
- ► Black tea is completely fermented

During the oxidation process enzymes in the tea change the polyphenols (the compounds in tea that make it healthy) into less active components. In green tea the process of steaming the leaves prevents oxidation from occurring. These polyphenols also provide many antioxidant and anticancer properties.

Flavonoids are the most abundant polyphenol in green tea. A flavonoid is one of a group of compounds found in plants. There are more than 4,000 known flavonoids. They are responsible for the deep colors of berries and are found in some fruits, vegetables, nuts, seeds, grains, legumes, coffee, wine, and of course, tea. Flavanols, also known as catechins, are a type of flavonoid that has received a great deal of attention for its anti-cancer effects. Green tea contains about 30 to 40% catechins, while black tea contains only 5 to 10% after the fermentation process.

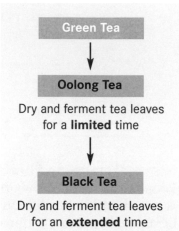

What about oolong tea? Oolong tea falls in between green and black tea in terms of the compounds it contains. Its benefits also fall somewhere between those of green and black tea. The major drawback to oolong tea is that it may be difficult to locate easily. If you wish to try it, check your local health food store.

Other Teas

Essiac tea was first used in Canada in the 1920s by a nurse named Rene Caisse. She claimed that she received the recipe for this herbal tea from a woman who told her it had cured her breast cancer.

The four primary herbs found in Essiac tea are:
burdock root (scientific name Arctium lappa)
Indian rhubarb (scientific name Rheum palmatum)
sheep sorrel (scientific name Rumex acetosella)
inner bark of the slippery elm (scientific name Ulmus fulva or Ulmus rubra)

Rene Caisse gave Essiac to hundreds of cancer patients, either by injection or orally in the form of tea. Over the course of time she changed the herbal mixture often. By 1938 Essiac was becoming fairly popular, although people had concerns about its use. This led to an investigation by the Cancer Commission of Ontario. They visited Rene's clinic and listened to testimonials from patients she treated. The investigation concluded that there was little evidence to support its benefits for treatment of cancer. Regardless, her clinic remained open due to public support, even though she did not have official approval.

Years after this report was published, Rene Caisse began to work with a famous American physician, Dr. Charles Brusch, in an effort to change the original herbal mixture and promote its widespread use. Their laboratory and clinical experience convinced them to add four additional herbs to the original recipe in order to make it more effective and to make it taste better.

The four additional herbs are:
blessed thistle
kelp
red clover
watercress

Caisse's original recipe is now manufactured and sold as Essiac tea. Flor-Essence tea, the eight-herb tea that Caisse and Dr. Brusch developed, is also available to the general public. Both are advertised as "health-promoting herbal teas" and are available through health food stores. Advocates claim that if taken during cancer treatments (i.e., chemotherapy or radiation) the tea boosts the immune system, increases appetite, and helps reduce pain. There are also claims that it may decrease the size of various tumors and keep patients alive longer. Most of the individuals using these teas today are doing so with conventional treatments and as supportive care for terminal disease.

Kombucha Tea
The kombucha mushroom, also called the Manchurian or kargasok mushroom, has been used in China and Russia for thousands of years. The kombucha is commonly referred to as a mushroom, but it is actually a combination of lichen, bacteria, and yeast. The kombucha is not eaten, but rather made into tea through a fermentation process. The daughter mushrooms, produced during the process, can be used to make more tea. This tea is believed to contain a number of nutrients and other healthy ingredients that may be useful in combating various diseases and may also provide a natural energy boost. Please keep in mind that these are only claims and that they have not been scientifically researched. Since it is made in such a unique way it may be difficult to find. Ask your local health food expert to locate either the kombucha mushrooms or bottled tea for you if possible.

Tea Facts
black tea—tea from fermented leaves
Ceylon tea—black tea produced in Sri Lanka
Darjeeling tea—black tea produced in the Darjeeling district of India
Essiac—four-herb combination tea (burdock root, Indian rhubarb, sheep sorrel, and inner bark of slippery elm)
Flor-Essence—eight-herb combination tea (burdock root, Indian rhubarb,

sheep sorrel, slippery elm, blessed thistle, kelp, red clover, and watercress)

Green tea—made with unfermented tea leaves

Gunpowder—a type of green tea exclusively made in China; the leaves are rolled into fine pellets that unfold in warm water

herbal tea—made from plants other than the standard tea plant, i.e., peppermint or chamomile

kombucha tea—commonly considered a mushroom, but actually a combination of lichen, bacteria, and yeast; it is converted to tea through a fermentation process

oolong tea—partially fermented tea

pekoe tea—whole-leaf black tea that has been flavored, such as orange pekoe

Common Natural Sources of Polyphenols (anti-cancer compounds):					
Beverages	Cereals	Fruit	Legumes	Nuts	Vegetables
apple juice	barley	apples	chickpeas	cashews	brussels
orange juice	corn	apricots	beans	peanuts	sprouts
green tea leaves	millet	black currants		pecans	cabbage
black tea leaves	oats	blueberries			celery
coffee beans	rice	cherries			leeks
cacao beans	sorghum	cranberries			onions
(chocolate or cocoa)	wheat	gooseberries			parsley
white wine		grapes			
red wine		grapefruit			
beer		oranges			
		peaches			
		pears			
		plums			
		raspberries			
		red currants			
		strawberries			
		tomatoes			

Grape Seed Extract

Grape seed extract contains a large amount of polyphenols—more specifically, flavonoids, and even more specifically, proanthocyanidins. Mixtures of these proanthocyanidins are called PCOs (procyanidolic oligomers). These PCOs, believed to contain a variety of health benefits, are found in many things, for example, red wine. They are also available in extracts from grape seeds, the bark of certain pine trees, and in the form of supplements.

Resveratrol and Alcohol

Resveratrol is a polyphenol compound found primarily in red wine and grapes. Lately, it has been the focus of much research, as have other compounds found in alcoholic beverages. This is because in a few studies moderate amounts of alcohol have been found to be healthy, and researchers are trying to determine why.

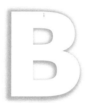

What the Medical Research Tells Us

Tea and Cancer

Epigallocatechin-3 gallate (EGCG) is currently considered the most important polyphenol component in tea in terms of cancer prevention. As we all well know, another component of green and black tea is caffeine. In fact, 1 cup of green tea usually contains 300 to 400 mg of polyphenols. Black tea contains about one-third the caffeine of coffee (35 mg), and green tea contains a little less than that. Fortunately, there are now green tea products you can buy that are decaffeinated. Additionally, the polyphenols are concentrated in these products so they contain anywhere from 60 to 80% polyphenols—the same amount found in the caffeinated teas.

A recent review of the medical literature on green tea seems to indicate that it can prevent a variety of cancers, although much more research needs to be completed prior to a specific recommendation.

So far we've learned that green tea polyphenols have shown greater antioxidant protection than vitamins C and E in a number of laboratory studies. Green tea polyphenols may offer protection from cancer by potentially blocking the formation of cancer-causing compounds such as nitrosamines. Drinking green tea with meals may inhibit these nitrosamines. (Nitrosamines are produced when nitrites, found in such foods as bacon and ham, bind to other products.) The popular practice of drinking green tea with meals is believed to be a major reason for the lower cancer rate in Japan.

Cancers that appear the most likely to be prevented by green tea consumption are cancers of the gastrointestinal tract, breast cancer, and possibly prostate cancer.

Remember that tea is a diuretic and can cause you to urinate more often, thereby losing bodily fluids (water). So, drink plenty of water if you drink tea so that you do not become dehydrated.

Green Tea and Cancer Chemotherapy

A few interesting studies have recently been published on the use of nutrition to enhance drugs used during cancer chemotherapy. For example, a recent animal study published in *Clinical Cancer Research* (January, 1998) was done on the effect of green tea (taken orally) and a common cancer chemotherapy drug, doxorubicin (also known as adriamycin). It was found that green tea enhanced (by 2.5 times) the inhibitory effects of doxorubicin on tumor growth. In fact, the doxorubicin concentration inside the tumor was increased with the green tea combination (in laboratory studies), but it was not increased in normal cells. The researchers concluded that drinking green tea may assist cancer chemotherapy drugs.

Doxorubicin causes considerable toxic effects to other normal organs, like the heart, although in the future, because of the antioxidants in green tea, it may be given to cancer patients to reduce side effects and improve delivery of drugs to a cancer.

Tea and Prostate Cancer

Population studies from Asian countries with a high consumption of tea indicate that cancer rates, including that of prostate cancer, are low. Japan and China, where green tea is regularly consumed, have some of the lowest rates of prostate cancer in the world.

A number of laboratory studies have focused attention on the different polyphenols—specifically, catechins—in tea. Early results are impressive. For example, EGCG (mentioned earlier in this chapter) has been shown in the laboratory to kill cancer cells. It causes these cells to "commit suicide"—a condition known as apoptosis—and at the same time healthy cells of the body are not harmed. Researchers have tested EGCG on prostate cancer cells and found that 1 cup of green tea contains between 100 mg and 200 mg of EGCG—a large quantity compared to other foods and beverages. In the laboratory, EGCG has also been shown to inhibit an enzyme called urokinase, which is needed for cancer growth. EGCG attaches itself to the urokinase and does not allow it to help a cancer grow and spread.

Animal studies have shown that the injection of 1 mg of EGCG, beginning two weeks after the injection of hormone-dependent and hormone-independent human prostate cancer cells, reduced the size of the initial tumor by 20 to 30%. Human studies have found that EGCG is well concentrated in a variety of body organs. One study found that EGCG is a strong inhibitor of the enzyme 5-alpha reductase, which converts testosterone into DHT (a more potent form of testosterone). Populations with lower levels of 5-alpha reductase also seem to have lower rates of prostate cancer. In fact, the largest clinical study currently being conducted (The Prostate Cancer Prevention Trial) to determine whether a drug can lower the risk of prostate cancer works by inhibiting this enzyme.

Please keep in mind that black tea contains a lower amount of the beneficial anti-prostate cancer compounds than green tea. However, there are compounds in black tea that are not found in green tea—such as theaflavins and thearubigins—that have not been researched in regard to prostate cancer. A few population studies (men of Japanese ancestry) have shown a slightly decreased risk of prostate cancer among men who consume black tea regularly. It is very important to pay close attention to future research results on both green and black tea.

Green Tea Supplements
Current research supports the use of natural green tea, rather than green tea supplements. Tea contains all the potentially beneficial compounds found in tea leaves, while supplements do not.

Essiac and Flor-Essence Tea and Cancer
It is very difficult to find any formal cancer studies, either laboratory or clinical, on Essiac tea. Beginning in 1959, and again from 1973 to 1976, Rene Caisse and Dr. Brusch requested that studies on Essiac and Flor-Essence teas be conducted by Memorial Sloan Kettering in New York. However, because of some difficulties in the setup of these studies, they were never fully completed. Preliminary research demonstrated limited biological activity, but specific conclusions were never

made. For the most part, the only evidence of its effect is from individual testimonies.

Between 1978 and 1982, The Department of National Health and Welfare (in Canada) reviewed data from 87 patients who were advised by their doctors to take Essiac tea for compassionate reasons. There was no evidence of improved survival.

While there have been no formal studies or controlled clinical trials on the use of Essiac in cancer, there have been separate and limited studies on some of the individual herbs found in these teas.

For instance, burdock root and Indian rhubarb, both found in Essiac and Flor-Essence, are known in folk medicine as a treatment for cancer, among other things. They contain a high concentration of flavones, tannins, anthraquinones, and some sugars that have shown limited antioxidant and other potential health benefits. In fact, a number of compounds are derived from anthraquinones, such as adriamycin (doxorubicin) which is commonly used in cancer chemotherapy. Burdock has also been shown to potentially cause cell death in some tumors. Extracts of Indian rhubarb have also demonstrated some of these same anticancer effects.

Slippery elm, another herb in these teas, is also known as a folk remedy for a number of health problems. It can be purchased in health food stores in a variety of forms. Compounds similar to the ones found in slippery elm have shown some anticancer activity.

There is very little information available on the herb found in these teas known as sheep sorrel, but keep in mind that most of the herbs used in Essiac and Flor-Essence have very limited published work.

Red clover, also found in Flor-Essence tea, has demonstrated significant estrogenic qualities in the laboratory. In a recently published study it was reported that a patient in Australia took red clover before surgery to remove his prostate. When his prostate was later analyzed it was found to contain some areas of cancer cell death, which the authors of the paper believed could be attributed to the red clover.

Side effects from Flor-Essence Tea have not been published.
However, these and other teas should NEVER be injected.

Recently, a death was reported when a doctor injected a patient with Essiac tea. If you have cancer and your doctor or anyone else wants to inject you with any alternative medicine, please get another opinion first.

Apart from a possible laxative effect or allergic reaction, these herbal combinations taken orally, as instructed, seem to be safe.

Kombucha Tea

This is an easy one. There have only been a few reports of side effects with this tea. These have occurred primarily among people who make their own version of kombucha tea. A survey indicated that in a few cases these home-cultivated varieties contained contamination from other microorganisms. However, the FDA has evaluated commercial producers of kombucha mushrooms and has found no dangerous organisms or hygiene problems. If you like kombucha tea, I recommend you buy it from the store rather than making it yourself.

Grape Seed Extract, other Polyphenols and Prostate Cancer

A recent laboratory study from the University of Nebraska showed that a grape seed extract supplement inhibited the growth of a number of different cancers. One of the tissues tested was from breast cancer and another was from a normal breast. The interesting thing was that it decreased the growth of the breast cancer and increased the growth of the normal breast tissue. Then, another grape seed extract was tested in the laboratory at the University of Michigan against a prostate cancer and normal prostate tissue. The same results were found. The more grape seed extract added, the more the growth of the prostate cancer was inhibited and the more the normal prostate cells grew.

The results of these preliminary studies are very interesting. However, much more testing needs to be conducted before a specific recommendation can be made. In the meantime, eating grapes is always a safe bet!

Resveratrol

Resveratrol, a polyphenol, is commonly found in grapes and wine, especially red wine. Laboratory studies have recently shown that it may help decrease PSA secretion and inhibit the growth of hormone-sensitive and hormone-insensitive prostate cancer cells. Again, far more research needs to be conducted with both animals and humans before specific recommendations are made.

In the meantime, there have been a number of studies that have shown that moderate wine or alcohol consumption may protect you against heart disease, by increasing your HDL (the good cholesterol), for example. There has never been a strong connection made between alcohol consumption and prostate cancer risk or progression. Even among men who were found to consume 57 or more drinks a week (a drink being equal to a glass of wine, beer, or shot of whiskey) for more than 10 years, there was no additional risk. The only slight risk was for men who consumed 120 drinks a week!

What We Believe

► Some alcoholic drinks, such as red wine, contain compounds that may inhibit the growth of prostate cancer cells, and may be estrogenic.

► A variety of alcoholic drinks contain a decent amount of polyphenols, which have been shown in the laboratory and in clinical trials to have anti-cancer effects.

► Most studies show no relation between alcohol consumption and prostate cancer risk or progression, even among individuals who consume 57 or more drinks a week!

► A recent study of wine consumption among Danish men and women was associated with a higher intake of fruit, fish, vegetables, salad, and olive oil. Researchers concluded that "wine drinking was associated with an intake of a healthy diet." (Tjonneland, A., et al., *American Journal of Clinical Nutrition* 69:49-54, 1999)

► Numerous previous studies have shown a link between moderate alcohol consumption and a decreased risk of heart disease.

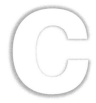

Bottom Line on Tea

Cost—Inexpensive

Green, black, or herbal teas generally cost somewhere from $3 to $10 for 24 bags. Essiac, Flor-Essence, and other specialty teas may run more, but they are still fairly inexpensive.

Dosage and Type

A good starting place is to incorporate at least 1 cup of green tea into your daily diet.

I do not recommend the green tea supplement at this time. Neither Essiac nor Flor-Essence should be substituted for green tea. I do not recommend kombucha tea for now either.

Side Effects

May behave as a diuretic. Drink plenty of water whenever you drink tea. If caffeine keeps you awake, try a decaffeinated tea. Green tea also contains a large amount of vitamin K, which helps the blood to clot effectively. If you are taking a prescribed anticoagulant (Warfarin), please talk to your doctor.

Green Tea—The Bottom Line

For the Prevention or Recurrence of Prostate Cancer—YES
For Localized Prostate Cancer—MAYBE
For Advanced Prostate Cancer—MAYBE
During Chemotherapy for Advanced Prostate Cancer—MAYBE

Green tea should be your first choice. Begin by drinking at least 1 cup a day.

15

Vitamin C

In this chapter:

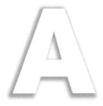

What is Vitamin C?

What the Medical Research Tells Us

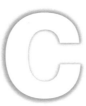

Bottom Line on Vitamin C

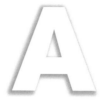

What is Vitamin C?

Vitamin C, first identified in 1928, is one of the most talked about vitamins of our time. Most of its fame originated when it was discovered as a cure for scurvy. It is water-soluble and easily absorbed. Vitamin C is not stored in large amounts in the body, although this does not mean that excess quantities are harmless. While most animals are able to manufacture their own vitamin C, humans cannot. Vitamin C is sometimes referred to as ascorbic acid.

Food	Vitamin C Amount (mg per 3.5 ounce or 100 gram serving)	Food	Vitamin C Amount (mg per 3.5 ounce or 100 gram serving)
red chili peppers	375	grapefruit and grapefruit juice	40
guavas	250	elderberries	35
red sweet peppers	200	liver	35
kale	175	turnips	35
parsley	175	mangoes	35
collard greens	150	asparagus	35
turnip greens	140	cantaloupe	35
green sweet peppers	125	green onions	30
broccoli	115	okra	30
brussels sprouts	100	tangerines	30
mustard greens	100	oysters	30
watercress	75	lima beans	30
cauliflower	75	black-eyed peas	30
persimmons	65	soybeans	30
red cabbage	60	green peas	25
strawberries	60	radishes	25
papayas	55	raspberries	25
spinach	50	squash	25
oranges and orange juice	50	loganberries	25
cabbage	45	honeydew melons	25
lemon juice	45	tomatoes	25

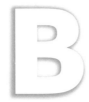

What the Medical Research Tells Us

Vitamin C and Cancer

Low intake of vitamin C has been related to a higher risk of nonhormone-dependent cancers. For example, cancers of the esophagus, oral cavity, and stomach, have been related to lower intakes of vitamin C. Although breast cancer is a hormonally driven cancer, a decreased risk has been linked in a few studies to a higher vitamin C intake. The generally accepted theory is that fruits and vegetables that contain high levels of vitamin C act together to provide anticancer benefits.

The Vitamin C Megadose Controvery

When it comes to treating cancer versus preventing it, the use of vitamin C has been entangled in major controversy. In 1976, Dr. Linus Pauling, along with Dr. Ewan Cameron, reported results that began all this controversy. They gave 100 terminally ill patients 10 grams (10,000 milligrams) of vitamin C per day. Sixteen of the 100 survived for more than a year. In the control group (patients who did not receive any vitamin C) only three patients out of 1000 survived for more than one year. Another study by Dr. Cameron determined that 10 grams of vitamin C taken daily by 294 patients increased their survival by 163 days (more than 5 months) compared to the control group. (There were 1532 total patients in the study.) These promising studies were controversial because they were not placebo-based studies. In other words, no one received a dummy vitamin C pill or sugar pill.

In 1979 and 1985 double-blind trials were then conducted at the Mayo Clinic and published in separate studies. In the 1979 study there was no difference in survival between the vitamin C and placebo groups. In the 1985 study, 100 patients with advanced colorectal cancer were given either 10 grams of vitamin C daily or a placebo. (The researchers chose colorectal cancer patients because this was the common cancer in the Pauling and Cameron studies.) Again, the vitamin C group experienced no advantage over the placebo group in terms of survival; in fact, there were more long-term survivors in the placebo group. So, there you have it—but the controversy continues. Many vitamin C advocates claim that the Mayo Clinic study did not, among other things, test a variety of cancers.

There is limited evidence that high levels (500 mg or higher per dose) of vitamin C can behave like a prooxidant. In other words, it may do the opposite of what it is supposed to do. Also, the basic fact remains that there is little change in the blood concentration of vitamin C from doses of 200 mg to as much as 2500 mg. So, more than 250 to 500 mg at one time probably provides little benefit. A dose of 500 mg of vitamin C is sufficient, and 1000 mg daily (500 mg at two times during the day) is the maximum for a 24-hour period.

The only exception to this rule is either right before or right after surgery. Higher doses (2000 to 3000 mg a day for approximately one week before and up to three weeks after surgery) may help in tissue repair, healing, and restoration of lost vitamin C during surgery and recovery. However, the data is very limited right now and controversial, please talk to your doctor. Try fruit smoothies after surgery—they are filled with vitamins and other nutrients. (Please refer to Chapter 21—Nutrition and Supplements During Prostate Cancer Treatment.)

Vitamin C and Prostate Cancer

There has never been a consistent relationship between vitamin C intake and prostate cancer risk. Some studies show a slight decrease in risk and others show that it has no effect. In addition, the potential benefit of vitamin C seems to require long-term usage at significantly higher dosages than the Recommended Daily Allowance (RDA = 60 mg per day). Most population studies in which men took doses of 60 to 100 mg per day from dietary sources (not supplements) have not shown a decrease in the risk of prostate cancer. Reliable data is not available regarding men who consume large doses of vitamin C from both dietary sources and supplements and their subsequent risk of prostate cancer.

Two laboratory studies have shed some light on the possibility of vitamin C having an effect on prostate cancer. In the first study a high concentration of vitamin C (along with a low amount of vitamin K) was applied to two different hormone-independent prostate cancer tumors. Researchers found that this combination was toxic against prostate cancer cells. In a second experiment, both hormone-dependent prostate cancer (sensitive to hormones) and hormone-independent prostate cancer (not sensitive to hormones) were exposed to high levels of vitamin C in the laboratory. A 50 to 90% inhibition of the prostate cancer cells occurred when vitamin C was added. Also, the hormone-dependent prostate cancer was more sensitive to vitamin C than the hormone-independent cancer. So, at least in a test tube, it seems as if prostate cancer is inhibited by vitamin C. Finally, when researchers placed human hormone-independent prostate cancer in mice and gave them vitamin C, their tumors were reduced.

Studies on the effects of vitamin C on prostate cancer will continue in the future. In the meantime, eat foods that are rich in vitamin C. They are good for you! There is no harm in taking a vitamin C supplement—in moderation!

Which Type of Vitamin C is Best?

The controversy regarding various vitamin C forms is about their absorption rate. In other words, the newer and more expensive forms of vitamin C claim they allow the body to absorb more of the vitamin.

▶ Ester-C or vitamin C from rose hips—These both tend to be more expensive than pure vitamin C. When tested against pure vitamin C supplements the absorption rate is about the same.

▶ Buffered vitamin C or sustained-release vitamin C—These are a good option for those individuals who cannot tolerate the acidity of pure vitamin C. However, they do not seem to provide any better absorption than pure vitamin C.

▶ Vitamin C with bioflavonoids—Only if the level of bioflavonoids is equal to or greater than the amount of vitamin C is absorption any better. If you are able to locate a supplement that meets these criteria, the absorption may be better, but the doses are so high it may also cause side effects.

▶ Chewable or powdered forms of vitamin C—These are normally filled with sugar and may promote tooth decay or an increased loss of minerals (like calcium) from the teeth. Stay away from these if you can.

▶ Pure vitamin C seems to be the best option. It is less expensive than the other forms and it is absorbed well.

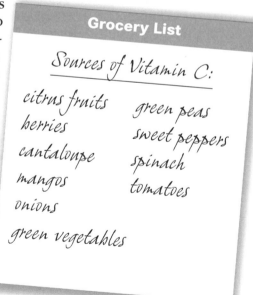

Grocery List

Sources of Vitamin C:

citrus fruits

berries

cantaloupe

mangos

onions

green vegetables

green peas

sweet peppers

spinach

tomatoes

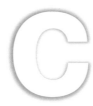

Bottom Line on Vitamin C

Cost—Inexpensive

Pure vitamin C supplements only cost a few dollars a month.

Dosage and Type—250 to 500 mg once or twice daily

Pure vitamin C tablets are your best option. Please take with a meal. Vitamin C's biggest benefit may come from the fact that it has been shown to interact very well with beta-carotene, selenium, and vitamin E. For example, vitamin C helps vitamin E to work in the body for a longer period of time.

Side Effects—Stomach upset

If taken in very large doses (thousands of milligrams at one time) it may cause diarrhea. Vitamin C is acidic and therefore may cause stomach upset (like aspirin) if not taken with food or around mealtime. If stomach upset continues, decrease your dosage of vitamin C.

Vitamin C Supplements—The Bottom Line

For the Prevention or Recurrence of Prostate Cancer—NO

For Localized Prostate Cancer—NO

For Advanced Prostate Cancer—NO

For a Radical Prostatectomy—MAYBE

> 2000 to 3000 milligrams a day (in two to three divided dosages) starting about one week before surgery and for three weeks after surgery. A few indirect studies suggest that high doses before and after surgery may help, but the data is very limited and controversial.

16

Vitamin D & Calcium

In this chapter:

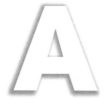

What are Vitamin D & Calcium?

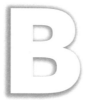

What the Medical Research Tells Us

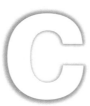

Bottom Line on Vitamin D & Calcium

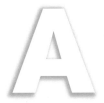

What are Vitamin D & Calcium?

Vitamin D

Vitamin D was first identified in 1920. It is a unique vitamin because it behaves very much like a hormone. There are two major food types of vitamin D: vitamin D2 (also known as ergocalciferol), and vitamin D3 (also called cholecalciferol—best source: the sun). Vitamin D2 is added to regular or soy milk and is the most common type found in vitamin supplements.

Vitamin D Sources:

► sun

Sunlight stimulates the production of vitamin D by your body. In fact, the sun is the best source of vitamin D. Only 10 to 15 minutes of general sun exposure two to three times a week in the summertime is enough for your body to manufacture a healthy amount of vitamin D.

► cold water fish

Salmon, mackerel, herring, tuna (packed in water—not oil).

► cod liver oil

Cod liver oil and several other fish oils are a good source of vitamin D. Please check the label prior to purchase—some also contain fat!

► Milk and Milk Products

In the United States, it seems as if milk is the primary source of vitamin D. There are several other good choices, as you can see from the list of sources, so don't rely only on milk!

► Multivitamin Supplements

Many multivitamins are a good source of vitamin D. Most contain about 400 IU per tablet. In addition, individual vitamin D supplements are a good source.

► Prescription Vitamin D—Calcitriol and Rocaltrol

The prescription form of vitamin D3 (Calcitriol and Rocaltrol) are more potent than vitamin D supplements. They are commonly prescribed for patients who cannot manufacture enough vitamin D on their own.

▶ **Other Sources**

Fish, egg yolks, butter, margarine, and dark green leafy vegetables are a moderate source of vitamin D. Otherwise, most vegetables are generally low in vitamin D.

Calcium

- ▶ There is more calcium in the body than any other mineral.
- ▶ Calcium is responsible for about 2% of the body's weight.
- ▶ Bones contain more than 99% of the body's calcium.
- ▶ Calcium is involved in many other processes of the body, such as heart

Food	Calcium Amount (mg per 3.5 ounce or 100 gram serving)	Food	Calcium Amount (mg per 3.5 ounce or 100 gram serving)
kelp	1100	peanuts	75
cheddar cheese	750	romaine lettuce	75
collard greens	250	rutabaga	75
kale	250	soybeans	75
turnip greens	250	wheat germ	75
almonds	225	artichokes	50
brewer's yeast	200	beans	50
parsley	200	black currants	50
Brazil nuts	175	cabbage	50
general multi-vitamin	150-250	dates	50
watercress	150	pumpkin seeds	50
buttermilk	125	prunes	50
figs	125	raisins	50
goat's milk	125	soybean sprouts	50
regular milk	125	carrots	40
sunflower seeds	125	cashews	40
tofu	125	cauliflower	40
wheat bran	125	celery	40
yogurt	125	cucumbers	40
broccoli	100	fortified soy milk	40
cottage cheese	100	oranges	40
olives	100	squash	40
sesame seeds	100	barley	30
walnuts	100	brown rice	30
apricots	75	sweet potatoes	30
miso	75	onions	25
pecans	75		

function and proper blood clotting.

► Calcium is mostly associated with dairy products, although there are many other good sources of calcium.

► Calcium supplements are acceptable when combined with healthy foods.

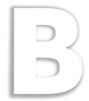

What the Medical Research Tells Us

The Twins—Vitamin D and Calcium

Before we continue, it is important to explain why vitamin D and calcium are both included in this chapter. Vitamin D has many functions, one of which is to signal the intestines to absorb calcium. So, if you are getting very little vitamin D in your diet then you are absorbing very little calcium. It is very important to make sure you obtain both vitamin D and calcium from your diet and possibly from supplements. This is why they are called "the twins"—they need each other in order to produce the maximum effect in the body.

Vitamin D, Calcium, and Other Diseases

A lack of vitamin D causes rickets (deposits in bones that result in abnormalities in bone shape and structure) in children and osteomalacia (increasing softness of the bones, which causes deformities) in adults. These diseases are rare today because most individuals obtain vitamin D from either natural sources or supplements. However, it was found recently that nearly 60% of elderly patients hospitalized for various reasons had inadequate levels of vitamin D.

Osteoporosis is a weakness in the bones, or actual bone loss. As men and women age they are at an increased risk for this disease, especially women. Most bone loss with osteoporosis occurs in areas of the body that absorb stress or weight, such as the hips, ribs, and spinal area. There are many possible reasons for an increased risk of osteoporosis. One is low intake of calcium.

High blood pressure has also been associated with a low intake of calcium.

Several studies have shown a reduction in blood pressure with supplemental calcium, while others have not. Results are inconsistent. It seems as if some individuals are sensitive to it while others are not.

Vitamin D, Calcium, and Prostate Cancer

Why is vitamin D important? Over 10 years ago a researcher from the University of North Carolina found that more individuals died of prostate cancer in the northern United States than in the southern part of the country. Researchers found that the same was true for both breast and colon cancer. Why? Keep in mind that it has been proven in the laboratory that vitamin D has anticancer effects. Researchers already knew that when the sun shines on your skin (limited exposure) it stimulates the production of vitamin D. Since the weather tends to be warmer in the south and people are outside and exposed to the sun for more of the year, it is possible that this continued production of vitamin D from the sunshine helps fight cancer.

Contributing Factors
► Age

Two things happen simultaneously when a man ages. First, there is an increased risk of being diagnosed with prostate cancer, and second, the ability to manufacture vitamin D from sun exposure diminishes.

► Race

Race also plays a part in the risk of prostate cancer. African-American men have an increased risk of being diagnosed with prostate cancer. This may be due in part to the fact that there is more melanin in African-American skin than, for example, Caucasian skin. Melanin blocks the body's ability to create vitamin D.

Asian men obtain more vitamin D from fish than Americans and have a lower risk of prostate cancer. Fresh tuna—a favorite of the Japanese—provides more than 16,000 IU of vitamin D per gram of fish. Wow!

► Location

Individuals living in the northern areas of the United States have more trouble making vitamin D from exposure to the sun. To further complicate the situation, even if you are exposed to the winter sun in these colder northern areas, the ultraviolet radiation from the sun is not intense enough to manufacture adequate levels of vitamin D.

Vitamin D is known to inhibit human prostate cancer in laboratory animals. What about humans? There have only been a few clinical studies in this area. Some have found that men with lower levels of vitamin D were more likely to develop prostate cancer, while others have not found this association. Other studies have found that the level of free vitamin D is what is important. Vitamin D is either bound to a protein called "vitamin D-binding protein" (also known as DBP) or it flows through the body freely. It is possible that the higher the level of DBP (the bound vitamin D) present in the body the greater the risk of prostate cancer. Free vitamin D is able to perform duties (anticancer) that the bound vitamin D cannot.

Studies have found that increased amounts of calcium intake may also be associated with a higher risk of prostate cancer. The body is sensitive to very high and very low levels of vitamins and minerals and tries to adjust each to a normal level. High intake of calcium may cause vitamin D levels to decrease. This is called a "feedback mechanism."

If, for example, the body has too much calcium, it responds by lowering the level of vitamin D in order not to absorb the excess calcium. This is a signal (feedback) to the body to reduce the level of vitamin D.

What if I take lots of vitamin D supplements? The problem with too much vitamin D is that it can cause hypercalcemia (too much calcium in the blood). This is a dangerous condition. Excess calcium may be deposited in blood vessels and organs, thereby creating blockage in these areas.

Remedies for Low Levels of Vitamin D:

▶ Vitamin D in Prescription Form

Calcitriol (Rocaltrol), the prescription form of vitamin D, is available through your doctor. A few clinical studies have been done with prostate cancer patients and the effects of differing levels of calcitriol. One study looked at this effect in men with hormone-refractory (hormone-insensitive) prostate cancer. They were treated with increasing doses of calcitriol (0.5 to 1.5 mcg). Only a few of the 14 patients had a decrease in their PSA. Most experienced hypercalcemia. Another study looked at patients with rising PSA levels who failed primary treatment for localized prostate cancer. In six out of the seven men studied the rise in their PSA slowed significantly with calcitriol (0.5 mcg increased to 2.5 mcg over time). One patient had an actual decrease in PSA. Hypercalcemia was a problem in this study as well. (One patient developed a kidney stone.) Three of these men had a stable PSA for more than one year. When the calcitriol was discontinued the PSA levels rose. Overall, these results are preliminary.

▶ Sun Exposure

Northern United States (or colder regions)—In the late spring and summer you should get 15 to 20 minutes of sun three times a week. You do not need to use sunscreen and it doesn't matter where on your skin the sun shines, i.e., face, arms, legs. Southern United States (or warmer regions)—Try to get a little bit of sun everyday during the warmest seasons.

▶ Vitamin D Supplements

Regardless of the area in which you live you probably need more vitamin D than safe exposure to the sun allows. During the warmer months 400 to 800 IU of vitamin D daily is recommended. A multivitamin normally provides 400 IU of vitamin D. During the colder months when the sun is not as intense you should get from 800 to 1000 IU of vitamin D daily from a supplement or multivitamin. Side effects begin to appear when the daily intake exceeds more than 2000 IU of vitamin D.

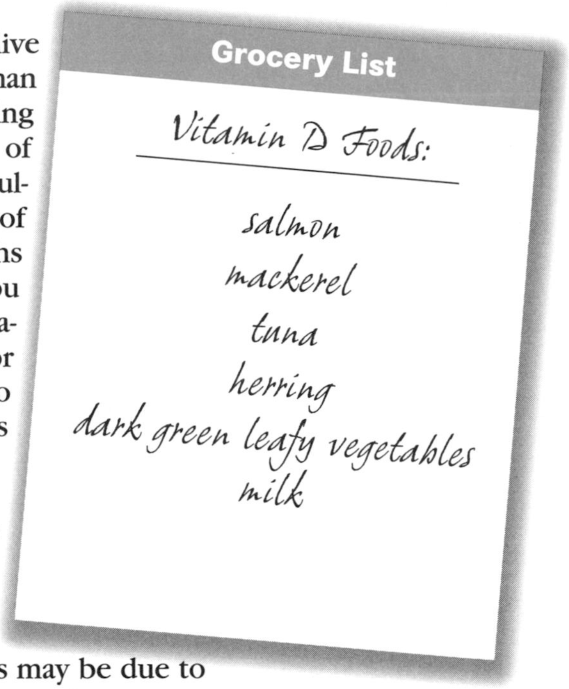

Grocery List

Vitamin D Foods:

salmon
mackerel
tuna
herring
dark green leafy vegetables
milk

Does a high level of calcium increase the risk of prostate cancer? Several studies have pointed toward an increased risk of prostate cancer with a greater consumption of milk and milk products. This may be due to the higher level of fat contained in these products.

▶ Consume milk and milk products in moderation.
▶ Drink either skim milk or soy milk.
▶ Prior to taking a calcium supplement, talk to your doctor.

Vitamin D and Chemotherapy

If you are undergoing chemotherapy for prostate cancer, talk with your doctor about vitamin D. A recent study showed that animals receiving chemotherapy for human prostate tumors had better results when given vitamin D than those on chemotherapy alone.

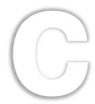

Bottom Line on Vitamin D & Calcium

Cost—Inexpensive
Supplements should cost less than $10 a month.

Dosage and Type
▶ Take with meals .
▶ Take 800 to 1000 IU of supplemental vitamin D daily during the fall and winter.
▶ Take 400 to 800 IU of supplemental vitamin D during the spring and summer.
▶ Do not take individual calcium supplements unless your doctor instructs you to do so. The amount of calcium in a multivitamin is generally safe.

Most multivitamins contain 400 IU of vitamin D. If your doctor recommends supplemental calcium, most of the research points to those products that contain calcium carbonate (also found in antacids), calcium citrate, or calcium citrate malate as the best sources. Some oyster shell calcium products contain high concentrations of lead—to be on the safe side write or call the supplement company to see how much lead is contained in their calcium tablets. If you are unable to tolerate vitamin D supplements, talk with your doctor about calcitriol.

You do not necessarily have to buy an individual supplement with combined vitamin D and calcium. These tablets can be large and hard to swallow. They can be taken separately and at different times of the day.

Side Effects—Excess calcium can cause a condition known as hypercalcemia.

This is a dangerous condition. Do not exceed recommended doses. Always take vitamin D and calcium, especially calcium carbonate, with or near mealtime.

Vitamin D and Calcium—The Bottom Line

For the Prevention or Recurrence of Prostate Cancer—YES

Take a daily multivitamin that contains approximately 400 IU of vitamin D. Walk in the sun for at least 10 to 15 minutes three times a week. Eat one or two servings of fish (stay away from fish oil supplements) weekly unless instructed by your doctor. You may want to increase your supplemental vitamin D intake to 800 IU during the fall and winter. Use skim or soy milk and products that are fortified with vitamin D. Inform your doctor that you are taking supplemental vitamin D.

For Localized Prostate Cancer—MAYBE

Take a multivitamin daily that contains 400 to 800 IU of vitamin D. Walk in the sun for at least 10 to 15 minutes three times a week. Eat one or two servings of fish (stay away from fish oil supplements) weekly unless instructed by your doctor. You may wish to increase your supplemental vitamin D slightly during colder months when sun exposure is limited. Switch to skim or soy milk and products that are fortified with vitamin D. Inform your doctor that you are taking supplemental vitamin D.

For Advanced Prostate Cancer—MAYBE

Take a multivitamin daily that contains 800 IU of vitamin D. Walk in the sun for at least 10 to 15 minutes a minimum of three times a week. Eat one or two servings of fish (stay away from fish oil supplements) weekly unless instructed by your doctor. Use skim or soy milk and products that are fortified with vitamin D. Inform your doctor that you are taking supplemental vitamin D.

During Chemotherapy for Prostate Cancer—MAYBE

Talk to your doctor about taking 800 IU of vitamin D daily, especially during chemotherapy. There is laboratory evidence that it might improve the effectiveness of chemotherapy drugs. Walk in the sun for at least 10 to 15 minutes three times a week. Eat one or two servings of fish (stay away from fish oil supplements) weekly unless instructed by your doctor. Use skim or soy milk and products that are fortified with vitamin D.

17

Vitamin E

In this chapter:

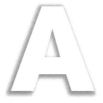

What is Vitamin E?

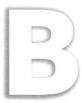

What the Medical Research Tells Us

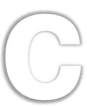

Bottom Line on Vitamin E

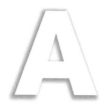

What is Vitamin E?

Over 75 years ago researchers discovered vitamin E. Since that time vitamin E has become one of the most researched vitamins. There are more than 15,000 published articles regarding vitamin E. Population studies and clinical trials have suggested that this vitamin assists with a variety of conditions, from diabetes to colorectal tumors to coronary artery disease. In fact, vitamin E levels are often cited as an explanation for the "French Paradox," or why the French live as long as or longer than individuals in the United States who consume an equal amount of fat as U.S. residents.

Vitamin E is a general name for a group of compounds classified as either tocopherols or tocotrienols.

Tocopherols	Tocotrienols
alpha	alpha
beta	beta
gamma	gamma
delta	delta

Natural sources of Vitamin E tend to increase fat intake. The best source of Vitamin E is a supplement.

Supplemental vitamin E comes from either natural or synthetic sources.

Vitamin E is assigned a small "d" to indicate that it is natural:
d-alpha tocopherol
d-beta tocopherol
d-gamma tocopherol
d-delta tocopherol

A "dl" indicates that it is from a synthetic source:
dl-alpha tocopherol

dl-beta tocopherol
dl-gamma tocopherol
dl-delta tocopherol

In general, vitamin E supplements are labeled as either "d" or "dl" alpha-toco-pherol. Acetate or succinate is sometimes added in order to increase the stability and shelf life of this compound.

The following conditions can decrease vitamin E levels:

► high intake of polyunsaturated fatty acids, which may promote vitamin E oxidation in the intestinal fluids
► high levels of vitamin A
► high intake of wheat bran
► high intake of pectin
► high intake of alcohol
► smoking, which can change levels of dietary vitamin E but not necessarily supplemental vitamin E

Vitamin E, Heart Disease, and Cancer

In the laboratory vitamin E has been shown to inhibit cells that may contribute to heart disease. It also has been shown to inhibit a number of different cancer cells in the laboratory (including breast and prostate). Population and clinical studies have provided limited evidence of an inverse relationship between vitamin E and heart disease and cancer. Normally, when a high-fat meal is consumed, the blood vessels respond by opening and closing, thereby increasing the chance that fatty deposits will clog these vessels. It is possible that vitamin E may keep blood vessels open and healthy.

Vitamin E and Prostate Cancer

Vitamin E has been shown to inhibit prostate cancer cells in the laboratory. In a recent laboratory study a concentration of vitamin E—used to suppress the growth of hormone-sensitive prostate cancer cells—neared the range achieved with supplements. A recent animal study also found that synthetic vitamin E inhibited the effects of a high-fat diet on prostate cancer.

A Finnish trial recently changed the perception of vitamin E's role in prostate cancer. In the trial, 29,133 Finnish male smokers, aged 50 to 69, were randomly assigned to receive either synthetic vitamin E (50 IU), beta-carotene (20 mg), both, or a placebo every day for 5 to 8 years. The men in the vitamin E group had 32% lower risk of prostate cancer and a 41% lower risk of dying from prostate cancer within two years of the beginning of the trial.

The confusion over vitamin E seems to be regarding proper dosage. It is generally accepted that 800 IU is safe for older adults without disease. No adverse effects on body weight or lipid and blood cell profiles are experienced at this dosage.

However, please stop for a minute and consider the following. If 50 IU of vitamin E (synthetic) was found to be effective (in the Finnish trial) in adequately reducing prostate cancer incidences and deaths, why increase the dosage? Until more studies are complete it is advisable to remain with the lower dosage, unless your doctor recommends a high dosage to treat a specific condition, such as hot flashes.

Gamma-Tocopherol and Prostate Cancer

Another common source of confusion occurs between vitamin E from the diet (foods) versus that normally found in supplements. Supplements generally contain alpha-tocopherol, while the typical American diet consists mostly of gamma-tocopherol. Gamma-tocoperol is commonly found in vegetable oils and products that contain vegetable oil, such as salad dressings, mayonnaise, margarine, nuts, and seeds. Alpha- and gamma-tocopherol are similarly absorbed and secreted from and into the intestines. High alpha-tocopherol supplementation (1200 IU daily) can actually decrease gamma-tocopherol levels.

Controversy does exist over alpha- and gamma-tocopherol and prevention of disease. The alpha-tocopherol concentration in the plasma is frequently used as a marker of vitamin E levels in the blood. There are studies that show an inverse association between plasma vitamin E levels and the incidence of heart disease.

The University of Michigan Prostate Cancer Research Center recently investigated the potential role of natural gamma-tocopherol versus synthetic alpha-tocopherol on prostate cancer. (Most of the previous studies examined the effect of synthetic vitamin E only.) Two human prostate cancer tumors were allowed to grow for 48 hours before both types of vitamin E were added. The first cell line was exposed to five different concentrations of synthetic vitamin E (dl-alpha-tocopherol) for seven days each. The second prostate tumor was exposed to natural vitamin E (d-gamma-tocopherol), also at five different concentrations for seven days each, although the concentrations were 1000 times lower due to the indication from preliminary studies of stronger activity with gamma-tocopherol vs. synthetic vitamin E. Both natural and synthetic vitamin E inhibited prostate cancer cells at all concentration levels.

However, natural vitamin E, especially gamma-tocopherol, demonstrated a greater ability to inhibit the growth of prostate cancer, and at far lower concentrations than synthetic vitamin E. It seems likely that gamma-tocopherol plays a role in lowering heart disease risk and possibly prostate cancer. As mentioned earlier, higher levels of alpha-tocopherol supplementation may suppress gamma-tocopherol levels. A safe dosage of 50 to 100 IU is therefore recommended for the present.

Synthetic or Natural Vitamin E?

Natural vitamin E (d-alpha-tocopherol) is absorbed better by the human body. Vitamin E with d-gamma-tocopherol or mixed tocopherols—d-alpha, d-beta, d-gamma, and d-delta-tocopherol—may also provide benefits. However, for the most part, synthetic vitamin E (dl-alpha-tocopherol) has been used exclusively in past cancer studies. Opinions vary regarding the use of synthetic versus natural supplements. My advice is to decide on your own, but keep in mind that synthetic vitamin E has been used in almost all of the clinical trials. Neither will hurt you— just make certain you take vitamin E on a daily basis. Natural sources of vitamin E are typically more expensive than synthetic. Pay attention to the results of future vitamin E trials for more information.

Vitamin E for Hot Flashes

Vitamin E has been effectively used by women suffering from hot flashes for decades. The University of Michigan conducted a small study with prostate cancer patients who were experiencing hot flashes as a result of hormonal ablation treatment. Patients who participated in the trial reported relief from hot flashes. This is one of the few times that higher doses are acceptable. Men experiencing hot flashes from prostate cancer treatment should take 800 IU of vitamin E daily, with a meal, in two equally divided doses (400 IU in the morning and 400 IU in the evening). Either synthetic or natural vitamin E can be used for hot flashes.

Vitamin E, Smoking, and Prostate Cancer

Several studies have proven that prostate cancer patients who smoke have a greater chance of dying early. The correlation between young smokers (under the age of 60) and death from prostate cancer is even greater. Vitamin E trials for prostate cancer patients who also smoke have not provided any conclusive results to date. It is advisable that you do not smoke under any circumstances. However, if you have been diagnosed with prostate cancer, it is vital to your health that you stop smoking immediately.

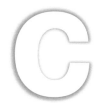

Bottom Line on Vitamin E

Cost—Inexpensive

Vitamin E supplements should cost only a few dollars a month. Natural vitamin E supplements tend to be a little bit more expensive.

Dosage and Type—50 to 800 IU

Use either synthetic or natural vitamin E supplements, based on your choice. Always take with a meal. Natural vitamin E tends to be more expensive than synthetic. Fatty foods are generally the best source of dietary vitamin E—so be careful.

Side Effects

May thin the blood, temporarily increase blood pressure, disturb the effects of prescribed anticoagulants or aspirin, and can increase the risk of hemorrhagic stroke.

These conditions generally occur when vitamin E is taken in high doses. Additionally, several studies show that vitamin E at higher doses (greater than 1000 IU) may act as a prooxidant. The men in one trial took 70 IU, 140 IU, 560 IU, and 1050 IU of natural vitamin E (d-alpha-tocopherol) daily for 20 weeks. The men in the 1050 IU group showed a decrease in their level of vitamin C over time, and vitamin E tended to behave more like a prooxidant in some cells.

There is also a possibility that vitamin E could thin the blood more than necessary. If you are scheduled for surgery please be cautious and discontinue use of vitamin E supplements one week before surgery and do not resume use until one to two weeks following surgery.

If you have high blood pressure or are taking aspirin or prescribed anticoagulants please talk with your doctor about whether or not you should take vitamin E supplements. Some studies have observed an increased risk of a hemorrhagic stroke with vitamin E consumption that could have been the result of higher dosages and their potential to thin the blood.

Talk to your doctor about the use of vitamin E and always take only the recommended dose.

Vitamin E—The Bottom Line

For the Prevention or Recurrence of Prostate Cancer—YES

Take 50 to 100 IU of synthetic or natural vitamin E daily in supplement form. An individual supplement is optimum. However, vitamin E from a multivitamin is also acceptable. Take with food.

For Localized Prostate Cancer—MAYBE

Take 50 to 100 IU of synthetic or natural vitamin E daily in supplement form. An individual supplement is preferred. However, vitamin E from a multivitamin is also acceptable. Take with food.

For Advanced Prostate Cancer—MAYBE

Take 50 to 100 IU of synthetic or natural vitamin E daily in supplement form. An individual supplement is preferred. However, vitamin E from a multivitamin is also acceptable. Take with food.

For Hot Flashes Due to Hormonal Ablation Treatment—YES

Take 800 IU of synthetic or natural vitamin E divided in two equal doses (400 IU in the morning and 400 IU in the evening). Take with a meal.

This is the only situation in prostate cancer where higher doses of vitamin E are acceptable. This dosage of vitamin E has been found to be safe and potentially effective for both men and women suffering from hot flashes. The results are preliminary, we are not sure if it works better than a placebo but, it is worth a try. If the hot flashes decrease in regularity or severity, or if they cease, decrease the dose of vitamin E being taken and wait to see if the results remain constant.

18

Zinc

In this chapter:

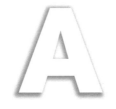

What is Zinc?

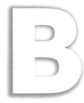

What the Medical Research Tells Us

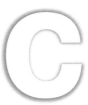

Bottom Line on Zinc

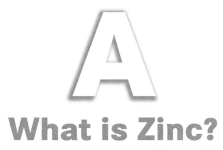

What is Zinc?

► Zinc, a mineral, is responsible for many functions in the human body.
► Zinc is present in all organs, tissues, and fluids of the body.
► The body contains approximately 1 to 2 grams of zinc.
► Nearly 90% of the body's zinc is located in the bones and muscles.
► The prostate contains a large amount of zinc.
► Zinc is necessary for the proper function of many enzymes and hormones in the body. Normally about 0.5 milligrams of zinc is lost from the body every day, but this easily replaced by dietary sources

Food	Zinc Amount (mg per 3.5 ounce or 100 gram serving)	Food	Zinc Amount (mg per 3.5 ounce or 100 gram serving)
oysters	150	buckwheat	2
general multivitamin (100% of the RDA)	15	green peas	2
pumpkin seeds (can vary)	8	hazelnuts	2
pecans	5	parsley	1
Brazil nuts	4	potatoes	1
split peas	4	turnips	1
almonds	3	black beans	0.5
lima beans	3	carrots	0.5
oats	3	garlic	0.5
peanuts	3	soy milk	0.5
rye	3	whole wheat bread	0.5
walnuts	3		
whole wheat	3		

Zinc is also found in all types of fish, shellfish, beans, nuts, seeds, whole grains, and meats.

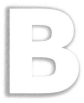

What the Medical Research Tells Us

Zinc, Prostate Cancer, and the Enlarged Prostate

The prostate contains the largest amount of zinc of all the organs in the body. Its role is not perfectly clear at this time; however, we do know three things:*

1. A normal prostate contains a certain amount of zinc.
2. A cancerous prostate contains a lower than normal level of zinc.
3. A noncancerous enlargement of the prostate (benign prostatic hypertrophy, or BPH) contains a higher than normal level of zinc.

Since a noncancerous enlargement of the prostate (BPH) contains a lot of zinc, it was thought that zinc was necessary for a noncancerous condition. In a few small studies zinc was found to reduce BPH. However, these were small studies and were inconclusive. It is well-known that in any BPH study the placebo effect is very strong and may be partially responsible for the beneficial results. A large and double-blind study needs to be done to prove any effectiveness for this condition. Regardless, there are many other effective ways of reducing BPH without taking enormous amounts of zinc (which may suppress the immune system and increase your risk of BPH).

A cancerous prostate contains a low level of zinc. In fact, this condition occurs early in the course of the disease. Is the answer to supplement with zinc? We know from research that zinc may increase hormone levels, thereby accelerating the growth of the cancer. Also, cancerous prostates have been shown to lose the ability to absorb zinc, unlike BPH prostate cells and normal prostate cells. What does this mean? Studies demonstrate that the decreased zinc levels seen in prostate cancer cells are not necessarily due to a decreased amount of zinc in the bloodstream. Prostate cancer cells do not contain zinc because the mechanism in

*Previously, researchers believed that zinc levels in the prostate could diagnose prostate cancer. The discovery of PSA to detect prostate cancer changed this theory.

the prostate that absorbs zinc no longer functions.

However, when zinc is applied to various prostate cancer cells (both hormone-sensitive and hormone-insensitive) in the laboratory the growth of these cells is inhibited. In the future it may be possible to use zinc for the treatment of cancer of the prostate if researchers can find a way for the cancer cells to absorb zinc.

For the present, obtain zinc from healthy foods and a daily multivitamin.

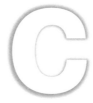

Bottom Line on Zinc

Cost—Inexpensive
It will only cost a few dollars a month to purchase multivitamins with zinc or to buy healthy foods. Do not take large doses of individual zinc supplements.

Dosage and Type
15 mg (100% of the RDA) from a multivitamin combined with healthy foods. Take supplements with meals. Do not take large doses of individual zinc supplements.

Side Effects
Unpleasant aftertaste, nausea, stomach upset, diarrhea, decreased immune function, and mouth, tongue, and throat discomfort.

In most cases side effects occur at high dosages. Do not take large doses of individual zinc supplements, and take multivitamins with meals to further reduce side effects.

Zinc Supplements—The Bottom Line
For the Prevention or Recurrence of Prostate Cancer—NO
Do not exceed the recommended dosage of 15 mg per day. Review the list of foods in Section A that contain zinc and make an effort to incorporate as many of them into your diet as possible.
For Localized Prostate Cancer—NO

Do not exceed the recommended dosage of 15 mg per day. Review the list of foods in Section A that contain zinc and make an effort to incorporate as many of them into your diet as possible.

For Advanced Prostate Cancer—NO

Do not exceed the recommended dosage of 15 mg per day. Review the list of foods in Section A that contain zinc and make an effort to incorporate as many of them into your diet as possible.

19

Alternative Therapies for Prostate Cancer

In this chapter:

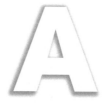

What are the Alternative Therapies?

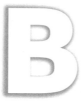

What the Medical Research Tells Us

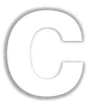

Bottom Line on Alternative Therapies

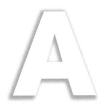

What are the Traditional Therapies?

A recent study examined various trends in alternative medicine use in the United States during the period of 1990 to 1997 and found it had increased dramatically from past use. Presently, there are more visits to alternative health professionals than overall visits to primary care physicians. Coverage of various alternative therapies has increased by a variety of health insurance companies and managed care organizations. In addition, the majority of medical schools now offer courses that cover alternative medicine therapies. Other countries around the world mirror the current situation in the United States. Studies have shown that at least one-third of some European populations and nearly half of all Australians partake in some form of alternative medicine.

Few studies have focused primarily on alternative treatments in relation to prostate cancer. There is a tremendous need for quality research in this area. Currently, the decisions a prostate cancer patient must make in regard to alternative treatment therapies are overwhelming. Hopefully, the next century will be the dawning of a new light for alternative therapy for cancer patients.

The Theory of Traditional Chinese Medicine

Traditional Chinese Medicine (TCM) utilizes various intervention procedures, such as acupuncture, herbal therapy, and lifestyle changes relating to diet and exercise. The cornerstone of TCM is the belief that the human body contains an energy force called "qi" (pronounced "chee"), which must be in balance throughout the body for proper health to be maintained. An imbalance in qi results in symptoms of unhealthiness. If the symptoms are not treated, this unhealthiness could progress to a disease state. Intervention by the above mentioned therapies is thought to restore imbalances of qi, thereby restoring good health. In order to maintain good health, TCM advocates moderation in diet and energy expenditures.

TCM, unlike Western medical science, does not label patients with a specific disease as a starting place for treatment. TCM bases treatment on symptoms, which describe the type and location of the imbalance of qi. There are different methods of categorizing qi imbalances within TCM. One of these methods is the "Eight Principle Diagnosis." The Eight Principle Diagnosis explains imbalances in terms of four opposing pairs of physical properties. Balance must be present within these pairs for good health to be present.

The Eight Principle Diagnosis Factors
yin/yang
excess/deficiency
hot/cold
internal/external

Yin and yang
Yin and yang are terms that Westerners have embraced; however, without at least limited knowledge in Oriental philosophy, the concept of yin and yang may be difficult for the Western physician to understand. Yin and yang are opposite attributes that complement and oppose one another. They represent the duality of nature, and encompass the light/dark, male/female, earth/sky, front/back, and up/down.

Yin Attributes	Yang Attributes
internal	external
cold	hot
nutritious	nonnutritious
storage-oriented	passage-oriented

Organs can be either yin or yang. Yin and yang must be balanced or compensation for one will occur in the other. Symptoms in either may appear similar but treatment therapies are very different.

Excess/deficiency
Excess/deficiency refers to overactivity or overproduction compared to under- activity or underproduction. Pressure in the body can be present due to an excess or deficiency of pressure. Excess pressure may be felt as increasing pain, while deficiency pain may be felt as constant less severe pain or even aching.

Hot/cold
Hot/cold does not refer to body temperature as measured by a thermometer, but rather to subjective feelings of body temperature such as the hot flashes

experienced by women during menopause or the cold chills of fever.

Internal/external

Internal/external symptoms can refer to changes in feelings of weight or heaviness.

The TCM practitioner listens carefully to all of the patient's symptoms, and by following the Eight Principle Diagnosis, as well as other theories, symptoms can then be related to specific organs.

> ▶ Yin/yang suggests the organ that is out of balance.
> ▶ Excess/deficiency and hot/cold are related to specific symptoms.
> ▶ Internal/external symptoms suggest the length of time of upset in the balance of qi.

It is important to remember that TCM does not assign disease names to symptoms in order to treat the patient. Therefore, there is no formal "prostate cancer" diagnosis in TCM.

A patient who is trying to prevent prostate cancer or who has been diagnosed with localized or advanced prostate cancer may not experience direct and overt symptoms but instead may be seeking immune stimulation or stress reduction. Acupuncture may be especially helpful in these situations.

Acupuncture

Acupuncture has been used by the Chinese for at least 2,500 years. It is currently an essential component of their health care system. The general theory of acupuncture is that pathways of energy (qi)—necessary for good health—flow throughout the body. Any potential disruption of this flow is believed to be responsible for illness or disease. An adequately trained acupuncturist is believed to be able to correct inadequate qi at various points close to the skin. This is accomplished by the insertion of needles and/or by applying heat or electrical stimulation at a variety of acupuncture points.

The scientific explanation that potentially accounts for the effectiveness of acupuncture is that by placing a needle(s) at a specific location(s) the nervous system may be stimulated to release various compounds—for example, opioids (compounds in the body that relieve pain)—in the muscles, spinal cord, and brain. These compounds will either change the perception of symptoms, or they will stimulate the release of other compounds and hormones that effect the body's internal regulating system. The body's natural healing ability is thought to be enhanced by acupuncture.

Meditation

Meditation is a means of contacting the inner energy that affects the natural process of healing. It involves taking time out from the world around you and calming the mind. Learning meditation can take a little time, so it is often best to take a class. There are several types of meditation: transcendental meditation (TM), mindfulness meditation and yoga. A meditation instructor should be able to help you decide which is best for you.

St. John's Wort

St. John's Wort (Hypericum Perforatum) is native to Europe, the United States, and other parts of the world. It grows in northern California and southern Oregon.

Hippocrates used it to treat many different diseases. Recent evidence has shown that it may have some effect against depression.

Kava Kava

Kava kava (or simply kava) is a member of the pepper family. It has been used for thousands of years, especially in remote areas of the world, to enhance peacefulness and calmness. It is popular in Europe for nervous anxiety, restlessness, and insomnia.

Ginkgo Biloba

The gingko biloba (or simply gingko) tree can live for hundreds of years. It bears an inedible fruit with an unpleasant odor. Gingko extracts are removed from the leaves and used to manufacture supplements. In China it is a sacred, cultivated tree and has been used for thousands of years to treat a variety of diseases and maintain proper brain function. It was brought to the United States in the late 1700s.

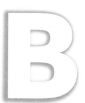

What the Medical Research Tells Us

The National Institutes of Health (NIH) issued a statement on acupuncture in November of 1997. According to this statement, based on several studies, the overall effectiveness of acupuncture can be considered legitimate. Acupuncture is most often used for acute and/or chronic pain relief or pain management. The consensus indicated that evidence demonstrates acupuncture's effectiveness for relief from postoperative pain and chemotherapy-induced nausea. They recommend further research in this area.

In addition, apart from the NIH statement, there have been a number of other studies that have demonstrated a potential relief from cancer pain through acupuncture therapy. This procedure may also help an advanced prostate cancer patient with pain control/relief due to metastatic disease and/or the nausea caused by chemotherapy drugs. There is also a potential use for localized prostate cancer patients who experience post treatment pain or discomfort. A localized prostate cancer patient may also seek a potential immune response from acupuncture. Acupuncture has been used with a number of patients with various malignant tumors and provided positive results in some cases.

How is acupuncture delivered to a patient with localized prostate cancer? According to TCM theories, the ear represents a number of different organ sites. A variety of needles are inserted into several specific areas of the ear to restore health to the prostate. Other common sites for prostate cancer treatment are the pelvic and abdominal regions. A patient with localized prostate cancer should expect to have needles placed in a number of regions of the body depending on the symptoms and the individual acupuncturist.

A patient seeking acupuncture treatment should keep a number of things in mind before starting this therapy. First, there are virtually no published studies to date that show the possible role of this treatment for prostate cancer patients. Side effects in general have been minimal in the hands of a well-trained practitioner. In fact, a recent report stated that forgotten needles is one of the more common problems. Severe side effects are possible if the acupuncturist has not received adequate training. Please check to make certain that your acupuncturist has been professionally trained.

Acupuncture for Hot Flashes

A recent small study from Sweden demonstrated the ability of acupuncture to potentially reduce hot flashes that are a result of prostate cancer treatment. Seven advanced prostate cancer patients who received hormonal ablation treatment also received acupuncture treatment for 30 minutes twice weekly and then once a week for 12 weeks. Six of these men completed at least 10 weeks of the acupuncture treatment. All experienced about 70% fewer hot flashes. Nearly three months after the treatments were finished there was still a 50% decrease in the number of hot flashes. Although further research needs to be completed, currently acupuncture may be a viable option for the treatment of hot flashes due to prostate cancer treatment.

Meditation

Meditation can actually effect changes in heart rate and breathing patterns, thereby reducing stress. As the mind slows and the level of tension in the body decreases, feelings of calm, peace, detachment, and sometimes joy occupy the mind, replacing tension. Meditation can help create a deep state of relaxation without loss of mental alertness.

In Chapter 6 the potential health benefits of melatonin were reviewed. As you recall, one of those benefits was a potential increased sensitivity to hormonal ablation treatment for prostate cancer. An interesting study of 16 women found that mindfulness meditation was associated with increased levels of melatonin. Further research needs to be done to test these theories. In the meantime, meditation is known to cause relaxation. Many cancer patients need techniques to assist with stress reduction.

St. John's Wort for Depression

Nearly 25% of advanced prostate cancer patients experience clinically significant depression. The number of patients with localized disease who experience depression is not known at this time. There are a number of options in terms of antidepressant medications. However, the use of St. John's Wort (Hypericum perforatum) can be considered for depression. Currently St. John's Wort has more proven beneficial research than any other herbal medicine. The potential beneficial components in this herb—hypericin and pseudohypericin—have been well researched, but the supplement's precise mechanism of action is still being studied. Animal studies have demonstrated that it has qualities similar to those of other antidepressants. Reviews of the effectiveness of St. John's Wort for mild to moderate depression have shown that it compares favorably with prescribed drug treatment. Research is limited for long-term usage and its effectiveness in more severe depression.

The safest plan is to purchase a St. John's Wort that contains at least 0.3% hypericin. Suggested dosage is 300 to 900 mg per day (taken in divided doses). Results can be expected in four to six weeks. Side effects are also less than those of prescribed antidepressants and may include photosensitivity, gastrointestinal upset, dizziness, restlessness, drowsiness, fertility problems and constipation.

Kava Kava for Anxiety and Tension

The initial impact of a cancer diagnosis can be very significant. Kava kava may provide temporary relief from this anxiety. Roots from this herb have traditionally been used for a variety of reasons, especially for their medicinal value. Kava kava is reported to have anticonvulsant, anxiolytic (anxiety relief), muscle relaxant, and sedative potential.

The active compounds in Kava kava that are thought to be the most beneficial are called kavalactones. A number of clinical trials have demonstrated that a kavalactone content of 70% may be helpful in managing anxiety and tension without affecting coordination, mental acuity, and other functions. Most clinical trials have used standardized preparations of kava kava containing 100 to 200 mg of kavalactones. Supplements were taken daily, either as a single dose or divided between morning and evening. Long-term use of higher doses (at least 400 mg) may cause scaling of the skin on the extremities. If taken as instructed, kava kava has been associated with few side effects. Please talk to your doctor if you wish to use kava kava to treat anxiety.

Ginkgo Biloba

Recent attention has been given to ginkgo biloba for the improvement of impotence or erectile dysfunction as a result of prostate cancer treatment. It is true that ginkgo extracts can improve vascular perfusion (passing of fluid); however, studies have focused on its use with either dementia or chronic cerebrovascular patients. No studies to date have been published on the use of ginkgo biloba for erectile dysfunction after localized prostate cancer treatment. The attention to ginkgo biloba stems from one study in particular with no placebo group. Sixty patients who did not respond to prescribed medications were treated with 60 mg of a ginkgo biloba extract for 12 to 18 months. Improved blood supply was observed by ultrasound after six to eight weeks in some patients. After six months half of these patients regained erectile function, and in a smaller number prescription medications were later successful. The study was followed by a blind, placebo controlled trial. Results published in 1998 indicated that no significant difference was found between the two groups (those receiving the ginkgo biloba and those receiving the placebo). This emphasizes the need for quality studies before recommendations are made. Several studies have suggested that ginkgo biloba may thin the blood; men taking aspirin and anticoagulants need to be especially careful.

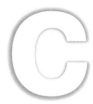

Bottom Line on Alternative Therapies

Cost—Varies

► Acupuncture therapy normally runs approximately $50 to $100 per session plus the cost of any herbs given by the acupuncturist. Check with your insurance provider to determine if any of the costs are covered by your policy.

► The cost of meditation classes also varies. Research several sources before registering for a session.

► St. John's Wort, kava kava, and ginkgo biloba average $10 to $30 each per month.

Dosage and Type

► Acupuncture requires several treatments to experience results for treatment of hot flashes.

► Complete at least one full session of meditation classes to obtain the maximum benefit.

► Purchase St. John's Wort that contains at least 0.3% hypericin. Suggested dosage is 300 to 900 mg per day (taken in divided doses) with meals. Results can be expected in four to six weeks.

► Kava kava should contain 100 to 200 mg of kavalactones. Take daily in divided doses or as a single dose, preferably in the evening. Results can be expected within a few days.

► Ginkgo biloba is not recommended at this time.

Side Effects

► Acupuncture—Possible side effects include forgotten needles, infection, and minor bleeding. Please make certain the acupuncturist has been professionally trained.

► Meditation—There are no side effects. Always practice meditation in a safe place and never while driving.

► St. John's Wort—Photosensitivity, gastrointestinal upset, dizziness, restlessness, drowsiness, fertility problems and constipation may occur. It should also be noted that there may be a potential for MAO-inhibitor-like drug interactions. Please do not use this supplement without first talking to your doctor.

► Kava kava—Long-term use of higher doses (400 mg or more) may cause scaling skin on the extremities. Please use only as directed.

► Ginkgo biloba—Not recommended at this time.

Alternative Treatments—The Bottom Line

Acupuncture—MAYBE

For relief of hot flashes due to hormonal ablation therapy for prostate cancer. Acupuncture may also potentially provide improvement of incontinence after localized prostate cancer treatment, and help reduce nausea associated with some chemotherapeutic drug.

Meditation—MAYBE

Meditation may provide relief for prostate cancer patients who experience anxiety.

St. John's Wort—MAYBE

For mild to moderate depression. Talk to your doctor if you are considering this supplement for depression.

Kava kava—MAYBE

For anxiety and tension related to prostate cancer diagnosis. Talk to your doctor if you are considering this supplement for anxiety and/or tension.

Ginkgo biloba—NO

Always talk to your doctor before beginning any alternative therapy on your own. Supplemental medicine should be a part of your written medical history. Keep personal records of your treatments, both conventional and alternative.

20

The A through Z Guide to Supplements, Alternative Medicines & Personal Choices

The A Through Z Guide to Supplements, Alternative Medicines, and Personal Choices

▶ Please do not use supplements or alternative medicine therapies as a substitute for medical treatment. Please discuss their use with your doctor and, if acceptable, use in combination with conventional treatment(s).

▶ If a specific dose is not included it is because a safe general recommendation has not been determined.

▶ Answers to whether or not the medical evidence supports the use of therapies are listed as: YES, NO, or MAYBE.

Alcohol
For the prevention or treatment of prostate cancer—NO
Moderate alcohol consumption has not been linked to an increased risk of prostate cancer. There is no solid evidence that moderate alcohol consumption should be stopped following a prostate cancer diagnosis.

Aloe Vera
For prostate cancer prevention and treatment—NO
For years there has been talk of the anticancer effects of aloe vera. However, the research is very limited, and it may in fact be harmful. It can actually delay wound healing after surgery; do not use the topical cream after surgery. It also contains high quantities of an omega-6 fatty acid (GLA) that has not been adequately tested in regard to prostate cancer treatment.

Alpha-Linolenic Acid (An Omega-3 Fatty Acid)
For prostate cancer prevention and treatment, especially from meat—NO (from flaxseed and canola oil—MAYBE)
Alpha-linolenic acid, commonly referred to as an omega-3 fatty acid, is found in many foods, such as, flaxseeds, hemp seeds, pumpkin seeds, walnuts, dark green leafy vegetables, red meat, soybeans, and canola oil. While a few studies have found an increased risk for prostate cancer due to an increased consumption of

these fatty acids, the majority of the studies have found no increased risk. Also, keep in mind that an increased level of omega-3 fatty acids from fish has not been found to increase prostate cancer risk. The bottom line is that if you consume omega-3 fatty acids from sources other than meat you should be okay. In the laboratory, studies have shown that omega-3 fatty acids inhibit the growth of prostate cancer, while omega-6 fatty acids seem to encourage the growth of prostate cancer.

Amino Acid Supplements
For prostate cancer prevention and treatment—NO

Amino acid supplements can be purchased in many forms. However, there is no research available in regard to their use for the treatment of prostate cancer. In addition, an excess amount of amino acids may be stored as fat.

Androstenedione
For the prevention or treatment of prostate cancer—NO

Androstenedione has been shown to increase levels of testosterone and/or especially estrogen. Therefore, in theory, it could increase your risk of prostate cancer or could encourage its growth.

Arachidonic Acid (An Omega-6 Fatty Acid)
For prostate cancer prevention and treatment—NO

Arachidonic acid, commonly referred to as an omega-6 fatty acid, is a building block for other fatty acids. It is found in meat and other animal products. Various cells in the body are sources of this fatty acid. Only a few studies have examined the connection between consumption of this fatty acid and prostate cancer risk. None have found an increased risk. It seems that omega-3 fatty acids inhibit the growth of prostate cancer, while omega-6 fatty acids encourage the growth of prostate cancer.

Astragalus
For prostate cancer treatment and prevention—NO

A few limited studies have shown that astragalus can boost the immune system by increasing the number of white blood cells. It can be taken in tea or capsule form. Until further research is completed, it is not recommended for treatment of prostate cancer.

Beta-Glucans (and mushroom supplements)
For prostate cancer prevention and treatment—NO
Beta-glucans, beta-1,3-D-glucans, beta-1,6-glucans, and beta-glucan from mushroom supplements are being trumpeted as immune boosters. Very few studies have been conducted in the area of prostate cancer. Please watch for future research prior to purchasing any beta-glucan product for the treatment of prostate cancer.

Bioflavonoids
For prostate cancer prevention and treatment—NO
Bioflavonoids are found in the skin of citrus fruits and brightly colored vegetables, as well as in supplements. Examples are: quercetin, luteolin, apigenin, and kaempferol. They are good for you and may increase the absorption of certain vitamins. However, there are no comprehensive studies on the effect of bioflavonoids on prostate cancer.

Black Cohosh
For prostate cancer prevention and treatment—NO
For treating hot flashes due to hormone ablation treatment—MAYBE
Native Americans traditionally used black cohosh to ease gynecological problems. Today, it is used in Europe to treat menopausal symptoms and as a natural alternative to estrogen therapy. It contains some plant estrogens. Women have had success with one or two capsules taken three times a day. If you have high blood pressure or heart disease or an estrogen-dependent cancer (breast, ovarian, or uterine) please consult with your physician before taking black cohosh. It may help men with hot flashes due to hormone ablation treatment for prostate cancer, although currently there are no direct studies to prove this.

Boron
For prostate cancer prevention and treatment—NO
For bone health from osteoporosis from hormone ablation treatment for prostate cancer—MAYBE
In general, fruits and vegetables are a decent source of boron. However, a few studies in women have shown that it may help prevent osteoporosis. In addition, it may make vitamin D more available to the body and reduce calcium loss. It is possible that men on hormone ablation treatment for prostate cancer may want to try a little boron, particularly if taking calcium supplements. Talk to your doctor.

Caffeine, Coffee, and Chocolate
For the prevention and treatment of prostate cancer—NO

Moderate caffeine and coffee consumption is not thought to increase the risk of prostate cancer. There is no evidence that you need to discontinue moderate use of caffeine, coffee, or chocolate after a prostate cancer diagnosis. Keep in mind, though—everything in moderation.

Calcium
For the prevention and treatment of prostate cancer—NO
For the prevention of osteoporosis from hormonal ablation treatment for prostate cancer—MAYBE

Avoid whole, 2%, and 1% milk. Instead, drink skim or soy milk fortified with calcium and vitamin D. There is limited evidence that calcium from milk and other dairy products (i.e., cheeses) that are high in fat can increase your risk of prostate cancer, although increased calcium by itself has been linked to lower rates of colon cancer and osteoporosis. I am not a big fan of calcium supplements for men at high risk of prostate cancer or who have this disease unless they have had hormone ablation treatment and need calcium to prevent osteoporosis. We do know that osteoporosis is accelerated in men receiving this treatment. Therefore, a safe dosage of 600 milligrams of calcium daily (no higher than 1200 milligrams) may provide help. Further research needs to be completed.

CENESTIN (soy and yam supplement)
For the Prevention and/or Treatment of Prostate Cancer—NO
For the Treatment of Hot Flashes from Prostate Cancer Treatment—MAYBE

Cenestin is a relatively new FDA approved supplement for estrogen replacement therapy. It is made from soy and yam. It may help menopausal women who do not wish to take estrogen replacement pills to treat their symptoms. There is a great deal more research needed, however, since it may help women with hot flashes, it may also help men who experience hot flashes as a result of prostate cancer treatment. Talk to your doctor.

Chamomile
For prostate cancer prevention and treatment—NO
For hot flashes and stomach upset from chemotherapy—MAYBE

Chamomile makes an excellent herbal tea. Chamomile tea may be used to ease stomach upset and menstrual cramps. It is being considered for future treatment of hot flashes and other symptoms related to hormone ablation and chemotherapy.

Chasteberry
For prostate cancer prevention and treatment—NO
For hot flashes from hormone ablation treatment for prostate cancer—MAYBE

Chasteberry has been used to treat hot flashes in menopausal women, and in the future it may help relieve hot flashes due to hormonal ablation treatment. A few cups of chasteberry tea or a few capsules can be tried for several weeks to determine whether it provides relief.

Conjugated Linoleic Acid (Also Known As CLA)
For prostate cancer prevention and treatment—NO

CLA has recently been proposed to help prevent or treat prostate cancer. Clinical studies are needed. Natural sources of CLA include beef, butter, cheese, and lamb, all high-fat products. Milk and yogurt also contain CLA and are far healthier choices. Please watch for future research results.

Dandelion
For prostate cancer prevention and treatment—NO
As a liver tonic for antiandrogen therapy for prostate cancer—MAYBE

Dandelion has been used as a folk remedy for liver problems for many years. Recent limited animal and human studies have shown that it may assist with liver problems. It seems to cause an increase in release of bile from the liver. It may be recommended in the future for antiandrogen patients who are experiencing liver problems.

DMSO (dimethyl sulfoxide) and MSM (methylsulfonylmethane)
For the Prevention and/or Treatment of Prostate Cancer—NO
For the Treatment of some types of pain from Prostate Cancer—MAYBE

DMSO and MSM (which comes from DMSO) topical creams have been used in veterinary medicine (MSM is also available in pill form, although it is most frequently found as a cream). However, in some cases individuals have used them topically on a sore spot to help relieve pain. To date there has not been a great deal of human clinical research in the area of cancer pain. However, preliminary data resulting from the use of DMSO or MSM for the treatment of other inflammatory or painful conditions is very interesting. Please talk to your doctor about these supplements for the relief of some types of spotty pain in the body. It is important to note that neither DMSO nor MSM should ever be substituted for pain medication from your doctor, but may instead be used to supplement your current pain medication.

Dong Quai
For prostate cancer prevention and treatment—NO
For hot flashes from hormone ablation treatment for prostate cancer—NO

This supplement contains some plant estrogen qualities. It is frequently used by women experiencing menopausal symptoms. There is currently no data that shows it relieves hot flashes for prostate cancer patients.

Echinacea
For the prevention and treatment of prostate cancer—NO

Echinacea comes from the purple coneflower. These herbs can be found throughout central North America. Almost all of the many different species of echinacea have a purple appearance, with the exception of Echinacea paradoxa, which actually has yellow flowers. The echinacea species most commonly used in supplements are:

Echinacea angustifolia
Echinacea pallida
Echinacea purpurea

Native Americans used echinacea more than any other herb for treating disease and injury. Since echinacea may contain an immune booster it should not be used by individuals who are receiving immunosuppressive therapy.
Few studies have been completed regarding its use for cancer. Until further studies are completed it is not recommended for cancer prevention or treatment.

Ephedra
For prostate cancer prevention or treatment—NO

This supplement has been blamed for a number of deaths. It is a nervous system stimulant. It is a bad way of losing weight and it is dangerous. Plain and simple, stay away from it. It can aggravate symptoms of an enlarged prostate.

Exercise, Walking, and Depression
To reduce your chances of disease and prostate cancer progression or related depression—YES

Two large and recent studies have found that walking (six times a month for 30 minutes or more) or a walking-related exercise have been shown to decrease an individual's chances of early death. Another recent study has shown a potentially lower risk of advanced prostate cancer among men involved in regular and vigorous activities, i.e., walking, golf, tennis, swimming, etc. Other studies have shown that moderate exercise may reduce testosterone levels in the body and stimulate the immune system, while intense exercise can cause immune suppression. Regular, moderate exercise is very important to good health! Several medical articles have reported that any type of exercise may help reduce depression. In fact, it has been found that exercise may be as effective as psychotherapy in some cases. (Although this does not mean you should substitute your psychotherapy for exercise.)

Fish Oil Capsules
For prostate cancer prevention and treatment—NO
For gaining weight for some advanced prostate cancer patients—MAYBE

Recently EPA, a fish oil, has been shown to potentially aid in weight gain for advanced cancer patients who experience weight loss from treatment. A dose of 1 to 2 grams per day is the amount usually taken. Please discuss EPA with your doctor if you wish to try it for weight gain.

Fructose
For the prevention of prostate cancer—MAYBE
For the treatment of prostate cancer—MAYBE

It has been found that among men who consume more than five servings of fruit a day the risk of advanced prostate cancer is lower. Interestingly, other fructose sources (soft drinks) also showed a decrease. However, it is also important to mention that individuals who consumed a lot of fructose from fruits also were less likely to smoke, were more physically active, weighed less, ate less fat, and consumed more fiber or fruits with lycopene.

Ginger
For prostate cancer prevention and treatment—NO
For the prevention of nausea from chemotherapy for prostate cancer—MAYBE

It is possible that 200 to1000 milligrams (or 1 gram) of ginger taken approximately 30 minutes before chemotherapy may help to reduce nausea. Ginger tea or ginger ale may work just as well. Ginger can cause heartburn and should not be taken by patients with gallstones. Ginger may also thin your blood (like garlic and onions), so it should not be used by patients on anticoagulant therapy without talking to your doctor first.

Ginseng

For prostate cancer prevention or treatment—NO
To offset fatigue from cancer treatment—MAYBE

There are many types of ginseng: American, Chinese, Korean, and Siberian. Ginseng is traditionally used to boost energy and prevent fatigue. Ginseng contains compounds called ginsenosides, which appear to stimulate a part of the brain, which in turn has an effect on the adrenal glands. Older studies support its use but newer studies do not. If you wish to use it for fatigue or energy, a common dose is 500 to 1000 milligrams, of which 5 to 9% is ginsenosides. Some recommend taking it for one month, then discontinuing for two months, and so on. Ginseng in higher dosages may be estrogenic.

Goldenseal

For the prevention and treatment of prostate cancer—NO
In the future for side effects due to antiandrogen treatment for prostate cancer—MAYBE

Goldenseal contains, among other things, the compound beriberine. There is limited interest and research in this supplement as an anticancer agent. It may also help increase the white blood cell counts of patients after radiation or chemotherapy. Additionally, it may be helpful for patients with liver problems or diarrhea caused by antiandrogen therapy. It should not be used by patients with high blood pressure. Further research needs to be conducted.

Hydrazine Sulfate

For prostate cancer prevention or progression—NO
For advanced prostate cancer patients with extreme weight loss—MAYBE

Dr. Joseph Gold, the developer of hydrazine sulfate, theorized that by inhibiting a certain enzyme it might be possible to reduce the problems of cancer-related weight loss. Through his research it has been determined that hydrazine sulfate may improve appetite and reduce weight loss. Dr. Gold has also reported that it inhibits the growth of cancers in animals. He has also tested it with humans, and now recommends it for all types of cancer. Dr. Gold stresses that hydrazine sulfate should be used in combination with conventional treatment. Further research and testing need to be completed on this compound. Please discuss its potential use with your doctor.

IGF-1 (Also Known As Insulin-Like Growth Factor 1)
In the future as a test to determine your risk of prostate cancer—MAYBE

A few studies have shown an increased risk for prostate cancer (and possibly pre-menopausal breast cancer) with a higher blood level of IGF-1. IGF-1 is a compound secreted into the blood by the body. Researchers are not sure if IGF-1 levels themselves promote the growth of prostate cancer or if they are simply a marker for an increased risk of prostate cancer. There is a possibility that this may be a standard blood test in the future

L-ARGININE
For the Prevention and/or Treatment of Prostate Cancer—NO
For the Treatment of some types of Erectile Dysfunction—MAYBE

L-arginine is a compound found in the body that can converted into Nitric Oxide. Nitrate Oxide can then go on to improve erectile function, although it has many other functions and does not always help improve erectile dysfunction. Several recent studies have suggested that L-arginine supplements in very large dosages (several grams daily) may help some men with erectile problems. These results arc preliminary and require more studies. Please keep in mind that many men experience erectile dysfunction as a result of conditions other than low levels of nitrate oxide. Talk to your doctor to determine if L-arginine may help you.

Licorice
For prostate cancer prevention and treatment—NO
For hot flashes from hormone ablation or side effects from antiandrogen treatment for prostate cancer—MAYBE

The root of the licorice plant possesses estrogenic activity. A special type of licorice extract called deglycyrrhizinated licorice (or DHL) has been commonly used for some conditions. Licorice root has been used in Chinese medicine for all types of things, including liver problems and hepatitis. It is also part of the herbal supplement PC-SPES used by some prostate cancer patients. Its estrogenic qualities may help with hot flashes from hormone ablation treatment of prostate cancer. Please talk to your doctor prior to consuming large amounts of licorice.

Licorice can cause hypertension and loss of potassium. Caution is advised. Do not use if you have had renal failure or are taking digitalis. Licorice can also lower testosterone levels significantly.

Mediterranean Diet, Macrobiotic Diets, and Cancer Prevention Diets
For prostate cancer treatment and prevention—MAYBE

Mediterranean Diet

The Mediterranean is filled with plant-based foods, such as fruits, vegetables, nuts, seeds, breads, beans, potatoes, and cereals. Moderation is recommended for meat consumption, dairy, and alcohol. Fresh fruit is a common dessert; olive oil is a primary source of fat; and garlic, onions, and other items are commonly used in recipes. The Mediterranean diet is also high in omega-3 fatty acids, low in saturated fats, and high in dietary vitamins (not supplements) such as the B-vitamins. Other factors related to this diet that are not commonly mentioned are regular walking and frequent social gatherings. Recent clinical studies (the Lyon Diet Heart Study) have demonstrated that this type of diet is associated with large reductions in incidence of early deaths, cancers, and heart disease. Whether or not this type of diet will reduce the number of clinically significant prostate cancers remains to be seen, but it is promising.

Macrobiotic Diet

There has been one direct study of the effect of a macrobiotic diet after a diagnosis of advanced prostate cancer (stage D2, or bone metastasis). There were 18 patients in this study, 9 of whom followed the diet for at least 3 months. The average survival time for the patients in the study was 177 months (more than 14 years), while the average survival time for the control group (the group of patients not participating in the diet) was 91 months (more than 7 years). Although this was only a small trial the results show hope for advanced prostate cancer patients. The only drawback is that a macrobiotic diet can be very difficult to follow. Please ask your local bookseller to locate books on macrobiotic diets for you.

Clinical Trials for Prostate Cancer

There are a number of clinical trials being conducted around the country for prostate cancer patients. For example, at the UCLA Center for Human Nutrition, 40 patients with prostate cancer who had a radical prostatectomy (with a Gleason score of 7 or greater) and an undetectable PSA after surgery were placed either in a dietary change group or in a control group. The dietary change group maintain a high fiber diet that emphasizes fruit, vegetables, cereals, grains and 40 grams of soy protein isolate daily. No more that 15% of their daily calories come from fat. Results of this study will be published at a point in the future.

Dr. Ornish is conducting a study of men with prostate cancer who have a PSA of greater than 4. All were either assigned to the experimental or control groups. The experimental group is on a low-fat diet supplemented with soy and antioxidants, moderate aerobic exercise, stress management, and psychosocial support. In the first year of this trial men in the experimental group experienced declines in their PSA that were larger than those of the control group. In men with initial PSA levels greater than 10, both groups experienced an increase in their PSA levels, although these increases were not as great in the experimental group. Results will be published in the future.

Other Diets

There are many other potentially healthy diets depending on your situation.

- Dean Ornish Diet
- Pritikin Diet
- Zone Diet—although you may wish to reduce fat intake to 20%

You can locate books on these diets at your local bookstore.

N-Acetylcysteine

For prostate cancer prevention and treatment—NO
For severe loss of muscle mass associated with advanced prostate cancer—MAYBE

N-Acetylcysteine (NAC) is a form of the amino acid cysteine. In limited studies it has helped AIDS patients who have muscle loss from their disease. NAC works like a building block for glutathione, a natural antioxidant. Some studies have suggested that it can increase life expectancy in AIDS patients. While no final determinations have been made, it may become an option for advanced prostate cancer patients who experience muscle loss.

Oltipraz

For the prevention of prostate cancer—MAYBE

Oltipraz is a drug currently being studied for the potential prevention of prostate cancer. Initial results have been encouraging for the most part. However, further tests need to be completed. A similar compound is found naturally in cabbage, broccoli, and cauliflower.

QUERCETIN
For the Prevention and/or Treatment of Prostate Cancer—NO
For the Prevention and/or Treatment of Non-Bacterial Chronic Prostatitis—MAYBE

Quercetin is one of many bioflavonoids found in nature. Recently, a small double-blind study was done with quercetin supplements. Men with chronic non-bacterial prostatitis received either 500 milligrams twice daily (1000 mg total per day) for 1 month or a placebo. Those who received quercetin had a significant improvement in their symptoms compared to the placebo group. Additional studies are needed to confirm this result, however, the initial studies are interesting. Several other small studies have also supported this finding.

Raspberry
For prostate cancer prevention and treatment—NO

Raspberry tea is helpful for menstrual cramps, pregnancy, and diarrhea. A few cups a day may help prostate cancer patients who experience diarrhea as a result of treatment.

Red Clover
For prostate cancer prevention and treatment—MAYBE

More information is needed. However, it is becoming clear from studies that red clover contains estrogenic qualities. It behaves much like soy and flaxseed. Dosage is unclear. Check with your local health store to see if it is available. There are a number of studies scheduled for the future. Please watch for the results.

SAM-e (S-Adenosylmethionine)
For the Prevention and/or Treatment of Prostate Cancer—NO
For the Treatment of Depression from a Prostate Cancer Diagnosis—MAYBE

Many people use St. John's Wort for the treatment of mild to moderate depression. However, a newer supplement called "SAM-e" looks like it may also help. These results are preliminary, but studies suggest 400 milligrams of SAM-e daily (or more) may relieve some symptoms of depression. Individuals with bipolar disorder (manic depression) should NOT take SAM-e because it may heighten symptoms. Talk to your doctor. Note: We are currently not aware of long-term side effects, if any, that are associated with this supplement.

Silymarin (Milk Thistle)
For prostate cancer prevention or progression—NO
For patients on prescribed antiandrogens—MAYBE

Other common names include holy thistle, lady's thistle, Marian thistle, Mary thistle, and wild artichoke. The artichoke is a member of this same plant family. Milk thistle is a naturally occurring flavonoid compound that has been used for years to treat liver problems. It has been shown in a number of studies to treat a variety of liver problems and to return liver enzymes to normal. Recently, a topical experimental form was found to protect mice in the laboratory from ultraviolet light and skin cancer caused by this exposure. From time to time a number of men who are receiving antiandrogen therapy for prostate cancer are forced to discontinue their treatment due to liver problems. It is possible that silymarin may help reduce or eliminate this toxicity. Silymarin is currently being clinically tested. Please talk to your doctor for more information.

Turmeric

For prostate cancer prevention or treatment—NO
For hot flashes from hormonal ablation treatment for prostate cancer—MAYBE
For liver protection during antiandrogen treatment for prostate cancer—MAYBE
Turmeric is a relative of ginger. Its key ingredient in medicine is curcumin, a strong antioxidant and antiinflammatory. It may also reduce high cholesterol by blocking its absorption. It is sold in both powder and capsule forms at health food stores. (The turmeric at supermarkets is usually not as potent because of its age and processing.) Take with meals, or add one teaspoon to a cup of soymilk.

Turmeric contains estrogenic potential, so it may reduce hot flashes from hormonal ablation treatment for prostate cancer, although studies need to be conducted. It has been shown to protect the liver from a number of dangerous situations. Hopefully it will serve as a liver aid during antiandrogen treatment for prostate cancer. In addition, turmeric has received much attention for some of its potential anticancer activities. Further research needs to be completed.

Valerian

For prostate cancer prevention and treatment.—NO
For stress, anxiety, and insomnia after diagnosis of prostate cancer—MAYBE
Limited clinical studies have shown that valerian may be useful for stress, anxiety, or insomnia after a cancer diagnosis. Please make certain any supplement contains 0.8% valeric acid. Recommended dosage is 150 to 300 milligrams per day. (Take it about 30 minutes to 1 hour before sleeping if you are using it for insomnia.) Use only temporarily (several days to a few weeks) until research provides a more complete analysis of this product. Please talk to your doctor first.

Water (Bottled or Tap)—No special preference right now for drinking bottled or tap water.

Over the past few years, sales of bottled water have increased by 400%. Today, more than one in five homes in the United States uses bottled water regularly. Is it necessary? First, there should be a focus on five minerals in your water for health reasons:

> ▶ Fluoride—important for strengthening bones and death. Fluoride in tap water has been associated with some major decreases in tooth decay and cavities in certain parts of the United States.
> ▶ Calcium—can lower your risk of osteoporosis.
> ▶ Magnesium—may be essential to proper cardiovascular function. Higher levels have been associated with a reduced risk of sudden death.
> ▶ Sodium—should not be consumed in large quantities. It has been associated with high blood pressure, or hypertension.
> ▶ Potassium—has been associated with a lower risk of stroke.

A partial list of bottled waters that can be purchased in the United States and their approximate calcium, magnesium, and sodium content is included. Fluoride content is not listed because it has been found to vary greatly from what is reported on the label. Few bottled waters contain potassium. Mineral content is listed as milligrams per one liter. (One liter is equal to approximately 32 ounces.) The RDA (recommended daily allowance) of calcium is approximately 800 mg. For magnesium it is 350 mg and for sodium it is 2400 mg.

Bottled Water	Calcium	Magnesium	Sodium
(mineral amount in mg per liter of bottled water)			
Adobe Springs	5	95	5
Alpine Spring	25	5	15
Apollinaris*	95	125	425
Arrowhead	20	5	5
A Sante	5	1	160
Black Mountain	25	1	10
Calistoga	10	2	165
Canadian Glacier	1	0	1
Canadian Spring	10	5	2
Carolina Mountain	5	0	5
Clairval	20	5	15

Contrexeville*	545	45	0
Deer Park	1	1	1
Evian*	80	25	5
Ferrarelle*	460	20	50
Gerolsteiner*	370	110	135
Great Bear	1	1	5
Henniez*	0	20	5
La Croix	35	20	5
Levissima*	15	1	2
Lithia Springs	120	5	680
Loka*	5	5	140
Mendocino	240	120	260
Monclair	10	10	475
Mountain Valley Spring	160	5	1
Naya	40	20	5
Ozarka	20	1	5
Passugger*	235	25	45
Pedras Salgadas*	130	2	500
Perrier*	145	5	15
Poland Spring	1	1	5
Pure Hawaiian	0	0	0
Radenska*	200	95	550
Ramlosa*	0	0	0
San Pellegrino*	205	55	45
Sierra	0	0	0
Spa*	5	1	5
Sparkletts	5	5	15
Sparkling Mineral	2	1	30
Talawanda Spring	0	0	5
Talking Rain	2	2	0
Tap water (from faucet)	85 or less	50 or less	195 or less
Tipperary*	35	25	25
Valser*	435	55	10
Vichi Celestins*	100	60	1,200
Vichy Springs	155	50	1,095
Vittel*	180	40	5
Volvic*	10	5	10
Zephyrhills	50	5	5

Indicates that the water is from Europe, while all others are from North America.

Several of the carbonated mineral waters (Apollinaris, Perrier, San Pellegrino) seem to contain higher amounts of minerals, including sodium, but there are exceptions (e.g., Ramlosa, which has no mineral content). The noncarbonated waters normally contain fewer minerals. Bottled waters from Europe tend to have a higher mineral content than those from North America.

Tap water generally contains a good deal of minerals, but this content varies widely from location to location. If you wish to determine the mineral content of your tap water you can have it tested in a laboratory, or call the water company, or have it independently tested (check the Yellow Pages). If you live near a waste site or industrial area it is advisable to have your water tested.

A frequently asked question is whether to use a filter for tap water. If testing indicates that the tap water may be harmful, or you like the taste of tap water with a filter, then buy one. However, keep in mind that it will probably also filter out important ingredients like fluoride.

Finally, there have been only a few studies of tap water and cancer risk. For example, in a study from Spain, gastric cancer rates were higher in men and women who had high levels of nitrates in their drinking water. It was also found that prostate cancer rates were higher in men whose water contained higher amounts of nitrates. Please remember that there have been only a few studies— no final results have been determined to date.

To have your tap water tested in your home, call the Environmental Protection Agency at 1-800-426-4791. Operators can direct you to a state-certified agency that provides you with a list of local testing laboratories. Cost for testing ranges from $10 for one specific contaminant to $400 for packages.

How about water filters? You can purchase water filters tested by the Water Quality Association (WQA): WQA, 4151 Naperville Road, Lisle, Illinois 60532.

There are three basic water filters: carafe filters, faucet filters, and reverse osmosis systems.

Carafe Filters

Carafe filters remove chlorine, lead, and some sediment. They do not remove nitrates, microscopic organisms, or pesticides. When tap water runs through the top, particles are absorbed by filter screens into an activated carbon filter. Cost is $25 to $50. Replacement filters cost $5 to $10 each, and must be replaced every one to three months. Carafe filters are available in pitcher or dispenser form and are the easiest way to filter water. They can be stored on the countertop or in the refrigerator.

Faucet Filters

Faucet filters remove chlorine, lead, and some microscopic organisms. However, the models can vary, so read the label to determine what they remove. These filters come in three types. The first type attaches directly onto the faucet, the second rests on the countertop and is attached to the faucet by a hose, and the third type connects directly with the cold water line under the sink. Carbon filters are used in combination with polyethylene for better filtering. The cost of these varies from $30 to $300. Replacement filters cost $15 to $200. Filters should be replaced once or twice a year. The under-the-counter filter requires the assistance of a plumber.

Reverse Osmosis Systems

Reverse osmosis systems remove chlorine, lead, nitrates, some chemicals, microscopic organisms, and salt. They can remove almost anything, including gases such as radon. Water is processed through two carbon filters and a synthetic membrane. Cost is $700 to $1000. Carbon filter replacements are approximately $50 each. The synthetic screen runs close to $100. The two carbon filters need to be replaced once a year; the synthetic screen needs to be replaced every three to five years. It will take up most of your under-the-counter space and it wastes three to five gallons of water for every one gallon of purified water. These are the most effective filters.

Weight (Healthy Body Weight)—YES

Increased weight can increase your chances of diabetes (type II), high cholesterol, and heart disease, and has been associated with a number of hormonal-dependent cancers, such as breast, ovarian, and prostate cancer. Individuals with abnormal weight of the upper body have also been found to experience unfavorable changes in hormonal levels. For example, the amount of sex hormone-binding globulin can be reduced by added weight, which means free testosterone levels can increase. In addition, there is recent evidence to show that other factors related to weight gain could increase prostate cancer growth. Regardless, there is little doubt that maintaining a healthy body weight is also healthy for you overall.

The following have undergone limited research. No testing has been done to determine their effect on prostate cancer. Further testing needs to be completed prior to their use. Please watch for their test results.

▶ Bilberry—for circulation

► Bee pollen and royal jelly for general health

► Benecol and Take Control margarine spreads to reduce cholesterol

► Cancell (also known as Entelev and Cantron) cancer treatment

► Carob (and bananas) to reduce diarrhea

► Cat's Claw for an immune boost

► Electromagnetic fields from power lines—as cancer causing

► Noni juice or supplements from the plant (Morinda citrifolia) from Hawaii—to promote health

► Octacosanol for fatigue

► Pregnenolone—which can be converted to DHEA, testosterone, and other hormones—may help combat aging problems (stay away from this)

► Qi gong as an exercise may be healthy

► Rosemary for cancer protection

► Silicon from high-fiber foods—for general health

► Thymic protein A—for an immune boost

► Wheat grass for general health

► Yohimbe for impotence

21

Nutrition &
Supplements
During Prostate
Cancer Treatment

In this chapter:

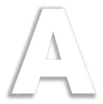

General Recommendations

Nutrition & Supplements During Specific Procedures

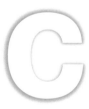

Summary

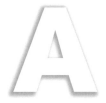

General Recommendations

One of the most effective ways of dealing with prostate cancer treatment is to remember the following:

Be mentally prepared and healthy about your treatment. Determine what will help you accomplish this goal and do it! It may enhance your chances of a positive result.

Do not be discouraged about reducing your supplements during procedures. You can maintain nutrition levels through eating healthy.

For years the National Cancer Institute has advocated at least five servings of fruits and vegetables per day. To accomplish this, my favorite recommendation is to drink smoothies! Smoothies can provide your daily servings of fruit, as well as anticancer compounds, vitamins, minerals, and fiber. All you need is a good blender with a tight lid and a "high speed" button. Drink immediately—the best nutritional value is obtained as soon as they are ready! Freeze leftover smoothies in ice cube trays. You can use the ice cubes in smoothies later.

The flaxseed and soy protein powder in each smoothie will provide plant estrogens and fiber. If you do not

Very Berry Smoothie

Contains more fiber than most "fiber-filled" foods. It also contains plant estrogens from soy and flaxseed. Combine all ingredients in a blender and mix until smooth.

1 cup blackberries
1 cup blueberries
1-2 tablespoons whole flaxseeds
1 cup sliced strawberries
1 cup low-fat soymilk
1/3 cup soy protein powder

Each serving contains approximately: 250 calories, 25-30 grams of carbohydrates, 4 grams of fat, 30 grams of protein, 10 grams of fiber, 300 milligrams of sodium, about 10% of your daily calcium, 5% of your daily vitamin A, and over 100% of your daily vitamin C.

Hawaiian Delight Smoothie

Provides almost a three-day supply of vitamin C and is a good source of fiber and potassium. Combine all ingredients in a blender and mix until smooth.

1 banana, cut into small pieces
1-2 tablespoons whole flaxseeds
2-3 kiwi fruit, peeled and sliced
1/2 cup mango, peeled and sliced
1/2 cup papaya, peeled and sliced
1 cup orange juice
1/3 cup soy protein powder

Each serving contains approximately: 300 calories, 50 grams of carbohydrates, 2 grams of fat, 25-30 grams of protein, 5 grams of fiber, 300 milligrams of sodium, 10% of your daily calcium, 20% of your daily vitamin A, and about 300% of your daily vitamin C.

Melon Melange Smoothie

Heavenly! Combine all ingredients in a blender and mix until smooth.

2 cups cantaloupe, sliced
1 cup honeydew melon, sliced
1-2 tablespoons whole flaxseeds
1 tablespoon lime juice
1/2 cup mango juice
1/3 cup soy protein powder
1 cup watermelon, sliced and seedless

Each serving contains approximately: 300 calories, 45 grams of carbohydrates, 2 grams of fat, 25 grams of protein, 5 grams of fiber, 300 milligrams of sodium, 10% of your daily calcium, 60% of your daily vitamin A, and about 200% of your daily vitamin C.

have time to make your own smoothies, you can buy them from your local health food store.

Note: Variety is the spice of life! Experiment with fruits and vegetables to discover your favorite smoothie. The addition of bran (1/4 cup), flaxseed (1-2 tablespoons), soy protein powder (1/3 cup), spirulina powder (1 tablespoon), wheat germ (1/4 cup), or wheat grass juice (1-2 tablespoons) provides you with fiber, vitamins, minerals, plant estrogens, and many other healthy ingredients.

Overall, Eat the Healthiest Possible Meals During this Time

One week before and two weeks after your procedure, you should eat in the healthiest way possible. Try to live with the following guidelines:

► Low fat intake—minimal meat
► Increase consumption of fruits and vegetables
► Fish—several times a week

Peachberry Protein Smoothie

This is my favorite! Combine all ingredients in a blender and mix until smooth.

 1 banana, peeled and cut into small pieces
 1-2 tablespoons whole flaxseeds
 $1^{1/2}$-2 cups orange juice
 1 peach, peeled, pitted, and cut into small pieces
 1 cup raspberries
 1/3 cup soy protein powder

Each serving contains approximately: 300 calories, 45 grams of carbohydrates, 2 grams of fat, 25-30 grams of protein, 10 grams of fiber, about 290 milligrams of sodium, 10% of your daily calcium, 8% of your daily vitamin A, and 200% of your daily vitamin C.

"Lotsa Power" Smoothie

I think carrot juice tastes okay, but in a smoothie it tastes great and provides you with "lotsa" beta-carotene. Combine all ingredients in a blender and mix until smooth.

 1-2 cups cantaloupe, sliced
 1/2 cup carrot juice
 1-2 tablespoons whole flaxseeds
 1/2 cup orange juice
 1-2 cups pineapple, sliced
 1/3 cup soy protein powder

Each serving contains approximately 250 calories, 40 grams of carbohydrates, 2 grams of fat, 30 grams of protein, 5 grams of fiber, 300 milligrams of sodium, 10% of your daily calcium, 200% of your daily vitamin A, and almost 200% of your daily vitamin C.

► Drink plenty of fruit and vegetable juices
► Alcohol—either limited or not at all
► Make certain your diet contains soy and flaxseed
► Drink several cups of green tea daily
► Avoid fast food meals—they provide little nutritional value

Also, talk to your doctor about taking a general multivitamin during this time (with B-vitamins, 400 IU of vitamin D and 400 IU of folic acid). It might also be a very good idea to talk to a nutritionist.

Make Sure to Include Light Exercise Every Day

Walk every day for 15-30 minutes one week before and a least two weeks after your procedure. Try to go outside and walk. However, if this is not possible, walk in the hallway at the hospital. Being out of bed and moving around will help you recover more quickly.

Sleep at Least 6 to 8 Hours a Night

Sleep is essential for proper immune function, for recovery, and for releasing beneficial compounds, such as melatonin. (Please refer to Chapter 6—DHEA, 7-Keto DHEA, and Melatonin.) This is one of the easiest things for you to do and one of the most important.

Keep Outside Stress to a Minimum

Let your body recover. Stay away from work and/or situations that increase your stress levels. This is important for your immune system. Read a book you have always wanted to read, and watch your favorite movies—especially comedies. Keep fresh flowers in your hospital room at all times, and when you go home take your flowers with you. Take photographs of your favorite people to the hospital and call them to chat while you're recovering.

Socialize, and Talk About What You Have Been Through

Keep communication lines completely open. Talk with your mate about your feelings and hers. Talk, talk, talk, and then talk again! Communication will help to reduce stress—both yours and that of the people closest to you. Keep a diary of your experiences. Not only will this help you to express your feelings, it may also be an important record for future friends and patients in the same situation. If you are religious, try to attend religious services.

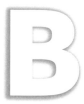

Nutrition and Supplements During Specific Procedures

Cryosurgery

Follow the General Recommendations in Section A of this chapter.

During cryosurgery, the prostate is frozen in order to destroy the cancer cells.

Very little is known for sure in terms of what to do before, during, and after cryosurgery. Stay away from supplements for the most part for one week before and two weeks after this procedure. It is okay to take one daily general multivitamin during this time. (It should contain 400 IU of vitamin D and the B-vitamins.)

Radiation

Follow the General Recommendations in Section A of this chapter.

Do not use any supplements for at least one week before and up to one month or more after radiation. (If you have temporary seeds or iodine seed implants that emit radiation for a longer period of time, your doctor may want you to stay away from supplements for longer.) There is very little data in this area, and what is available indicates that supplements may protect cancer cells during radiation. The free radicals that are generated during radiation kill cancer cells; you do not want supplemental antioxidants to alter this process. The same is true for proton or neutron radiation. **Talk to your radiation doctor** about taking one general multivitamin daily before, during, and after radiation and about supplements during radiation.

Radical Prostatectomy

Follow the General Recommendations in Section A of this chapter.

One week before your surgery stop all supplements, with the exception of one general multivitamin (with at least 400 IU of vitamin D and the B-vitamins). You may also take 500 to 1000 milligrams of vitamin C daily. Continue this process for two weeks after surgery (when the catheter comes out) and return to your old supplement regimen. (For example, reduce your supplemental intake of vitamin C.) An increased amount of vitamin C may enhance your body's ability to heal. The general multivitamin will most likely compensate for any nutrient deficiencies you may experience. You may not be eating much or at all right after surgery; stay away from supplements until you can eat again. Remember, surgery removes the cancer, so the use of vitamin C and/or a multivitamin should not affect cancer cells. You should not take any other supplements during this time; they aren't needed and they may make conditions worse. For example, large amounts of vitamin E may thin your blood, thereby creating problems during and immediately following surgery.

Hormone Ablation Treatment

Follow the General Recommendations in Section A of this chapter.

Your normal supplement plan should be acceptable during hormone ablation. However, to minimize side effects with this treatment you may want to consider one or more of the following options for symptoms of treatment:

Osteoporosis

600 to 1200 milligrams of calcium (and at least 400 IU but no more than 800 IU of supplemental vitamin D).

Hot Flashes

There are many ways of reducing this side effect. However, the top five are:

▶ 800 IU or 800 milligrams of vitamin E (400 IU in the morning and 400 IU in the evening). This is the only time higher doses of vitamin E are acceptable.

▶ Eat at least 1 or 2 servings of soy products and 1 or 2 tablespoons of flaxseed daily. The plant estrogen in soy and flaxseed should help reduce hot flashes. Try mixing 1/3 to 1/2 cup of soy protein powder or 1 or 2 cups of soy milk in your favorite drink. Tofu and whole soybeans are also a great source of estrogen. Drink smoothies!

▶ Limit caffeine intake.

▶ Limit strenuous exercise.

▶ Avoid very warm temperatures. An excessively warm room may initiate hot flashes or make them worse.

Other supplements reported to reduce hot flashes for women may also help men. They are listed below. There is very little research regarding any of these products, including proper dosage. Generally, one or two capsules daily should be sufficient. Please discuss them with your doctor prior to purchase.

▶ bioflavonoids
▶ evening primrose oil
▶ black cohosh
▶ blue cohosh
▶ chasteberry (Vitex agnus castus)
▶ ginseng (Panax ginseng)
▶ licorice (Glycyrrhiza glabra)—not the candy but the herb
▶ wild yam (Dioscorea villosa)
▶ Curcumin

➤ Red Clover
➤ PC-SPES

Finally, you may want to talk to your doctor about taking melatonin during hormone ablation treatment. The evidence is **limited** but points toward a possible association between remaining hormone-sensitive and taking melatonin (a few hundred micrograms to 20 milligrams daily).

Chemotherapy

Follow the General Recommendations in Section A of this chapter.

Apart from your regular nutritional and supplemental regimen, you need only consider one or two additional things during chemotherapy. Limited research indicates that taking 400 to 800 IU of daily supplemental vitamin D is important. Several animal studies have demonstrated a better response to chemotherapy when the animals were also given vitamin D. There is also limited evidence that caffeine may also enhance delivery of chemotherapy drugs. One to two cups of coffee or tea—especially green tea—daily are probably acceptable during treatment.

Other Treatments

If you are participating in vaccine, gene therapy, or any other clinical trial or experimental procedure, please ask your doctor what, if any, supplements are acceptable.

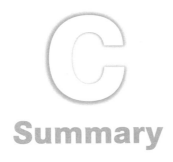

Summary

There is very little that has been absolutely determined as far as the use of supplements during prostate cancer treatment. The best thing you can do for yourself is to make certain you are in the best mental and physical shape possible. Patients who are physically and mentally fit have a better chance of not only recovering, but also recovering quickly. It really is that simple. Please follow the guidelines in Section A of this chapter.

22

Other Common Prostate Conditions

In this chapter:

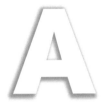

What are BPH & Prostatitis?

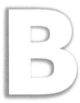

What the Medical Research Tells Us!

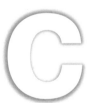

The Bottom Line on Other Common Prostate Conditions

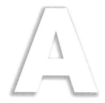

What Are BPH and Prostatitis?

BPH

Benign prostatic hyperplasia, or BPH, is a noncancerous enlargement of the prostate. As some men age their prostate enlarges. As it grows it squeezes inward, thereby restricting the urethra (the tube that runs through the prostate and carries urine). This causes an obstruction in normal urine flow. BPH can cause an increase in PSA levels.

BPH can be detected by:

▶ rectal exam
▶ ultrasound
▶ "free PSA test" or "free to total PSA test"

During the new PSA test two types of PSA are measured to determine the total PSA level.

▶ Free PSA—PSA that travels in the blood by itself attached to nothing, hence the name "free PSA."
▶ ACT-PSA—PSA that is attached to a protein.

Free PSA + ACT-PSA = Total PSA Level

It was recently discovered that many men with BPH experience an increase in their free PSA levels and a decrease in ACT-PSA. Men with prostate cancer experience the opposite.

BPH	Prostate Cancer
free PSA *(increase)*	free PSA *(decrease)*
ACT-PSA *(decrease)*	ACT-PSA *(increase)*

BPH is not necessarily painful, but it may cause some discomfort and, more commonly, abnormal urinary flow.

Prostatitis

Prostatitis is an inflammation of the prostate that is most generally caused by microscopic organisms or some unknown reason. It can cause pain in the groin or upon urination. It is not as common as BPH in older men, but the condition can remain for a long time. Prostatitis may also increase your PSA levels slightly.

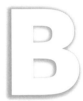

What the Medical Research Tells Us

Saw Palmetto

Saw palmetto is the most common and effective herbal treatment for BPH. Approximately 320 milligrams of saw palmetto daily (containing 85 to 95% fatty acids and sterols) seems to be the most effective for reducing the symptoms of BPH in the short term, and this dosage does not seem to affect short-term PSA levels. However, long-term studies have not been completed. Please keep in mind that there is a chance that long-term usage of saw palmetto may affect your PSA levels, especially large doses. Very few side effects have been observed from short-term usage: only 1% of men experience some erectile dysfunction.

If you wish to use an herbal supplement to treat BPH, saw palmetto is the best choice. Results can be expected in four to six weeks. Please talk to your doctor before taking any supplements.

Cernilton

Another effective herbal supplement used to treat BPH is Cernilton (also referred to as rye grass pollen). This supplement is slightly less effective than saw palmetto. The little research available indicates that a dose of 63 to 126 milligrams two to three times daily for 12 to 24 weeks produces the best results. Cernilton is not easy to find in the United States. Please contact The Cernitin America Company at 1-800-831-9505 for more information.

Pygeum Africanum

Pygeum africanum (African plum) is an extract from the bark of the African plum evergreen tree. It is used widely in Europe. Very few studies have been conducted on this supplement in the United States. Common dosage in Europe is 50 to 100 milligrams twice per day. The accepted content should include 14% triterpenes (which includes beta-sitosterol and 0.5% n-docosanol). The dosage is 50 to 100 milligrams twice a day.

Stinging Nettle

Stinging nettle (Urtica dioica) is widely used in Germany. Few studies have been conducted in the United States. Recommended dosage is 300 to 600 milligrams per day.

African Star Grass (Hypoxis rooperi)

African star grass is also popular in Germany. Harzol, one of the many types of African star grass, is the most widely accepted. It contains more than 70% by dry weight of beta-sitosterol. African star grass can be taken in doses of 20 milligrams three times daily for 6 months. Another popular supplement in Germany, called Azuprostat, has also been shown to be effective. African star grass is an interesting supplement to look for in the future. In a few studies it has demonstrated significant improvement compared to placebo groups.

Other Supplements for BPH

Pumpkin seeds (Cucurbita peopo), spruce (picea), pine (Pineas), and zinc do not currently have enough research behind them to recommend their use for treatment of prostate conditions.

Soy products have provided beneficial results for some men with BPH. Try to make soy a regular part of your diet. It's good for you!

Benefits of Herbal Supplements for Treatment of BPH

▶ alter the way the body deals with cholesterol (some cholesterol-lowering drugs help patients with BPH also)
▶ antiinflammatory effect
▶ antioxidant effects (by lowering the number of free radicals in the prostate)
▶ block receptors on the prostate that may normally increase prostate size
▶ change hormone levels in the body
▶ inhibit 5-alpha reductase (this is the enzyme that converts testosterone to a more potent form of testosterone)

Other Options for BPH

There are many possible options for the treatment of BPH. Herbal supplements are a good first choice for mild to moderate BPH. It is best to reduce caffeine and alcohol consumption and spicy foods.

What if herbal supplements aren't providing enough relief? There are a number of prescription medications that work by either shrinking or relaxing the prostate. There are also a number of outpatient procedures that are effective in more extreme cases of BPH.

Prostatitis—Cernilton

The only clinically tested herbal supplement for prostatitis, particularly chronic nonbacterial prostatitis (not caused by bacteria) is Cernilton. It is an extract taken from several pollens and may inhibit an enzyme that causes inflammation in the prostate. Its precise mechanism of action has not been determined yet. In a few laboratory studies it has been shown to inhibit the growth of prostate cancer cells.

It normally takes three to six months to produce beneficial results. Recommended dosage is 63 to 126 milligrams two to three times a day. Cernilton should not affect your PSA levels unless your PSA increase was caused by the inflamation. It is available in the United States from Cernitin America at 1-800-831-9505 (or visit their web site at www.cernitinamerica.com).

Other Prostatitis Treatments

There is limited laboratory evidence that soy products may also reduce the signs of prostatitis. (Please refer to Chapter 8—Flaxseed and Soy.) Antibiotics may treat bacterial prostatitis (caused by bacteria), and sometimes sitting in a hot bath also helps. Talk to your physician about your treatment options.

Bottom Line on Other Common Prostate Conditions

Cost—Inexpensive

Supplements should cost no more than $10 to $20 dollars a month.

Dosage and Type

▶ BPH—320 mg daily (or two 160 milligram tablets) of saw palmetto for several months. Saw palmetto should contain 85 to 95% fatty acids and sterols.

▶ Prostatitis—Cernilton in doses of 63 to 126 mg two to three times daily for 3 to 6 months or an equivalent dosage 1-2 times daily. (Order Cernilton at 1-800-831-9505.)

Side Effects

▶ Saw palmetto—Approximately 1% of men experience erectile dysfunction. Long-term effects of continued use have not been determined. Stomach upset is reported in 5 to 10% of users.

▶ Cernilton—A small percentage of men, not more than 1 to 5%, experience heartburn or stomach upset. Take with meals to reduce side effects.

Other Common Prostate Conditions—The Bottom Line

For the Treatment of Mild to Moderate BPH

Saw Palmetto—YES

Pay close attention to results of clinical trials on the various other supplements mentioned in this chapter. Talk to your doctor prior to the use of any supplement.

For Chronic Nonbacterial Prostatitis

Cernilton—YES

Talk to your doctor prior to the use of any supplement.

Summary

Summary

The following guidelines—an overall review of *The ABC's of Nutrition and Supplements for Prostate Cancer*—are provided to help you incorporate permanent changes into your lifestyle—changes that may very well help you to either prevent prostate cancer or inhibit its growth. They are simple and easy to follow. Please keep in mind that many of the supplements and dietary recommendations are still being tested. I have given you my honest opinion on each, based upon the research that is currently available. Please talk to your doctor prior to the use of any supplements.

1. Diet

► A diet high in plant estrogens appears to offer protection against prostate cancer. Soy products should be consumed on a daily basis. Soybeans, soy protein powder, tofu, tempeh, and soy milk are the best sources. At least one serving per day is recommended. The easiest to obtain and to incorporate into your daily diet are soy protein powder (1/3 cup) and 8 to 12 ounces of soy milk. Keep in mind that soy milk does not contain as much plant estrogen as soy protein powder.

► Another source of plant estrogen is flaxseed. Try to take 1 or 2 tablespoons of whole flaxseed daily. It can be swallowed with water, or ground and mixed into a beverage, sauce, salad, or smoothie. Flaxseed is a major source of fiber and omega-3 fatty acids. Avoid flaxseed oil, powders, and capsules until more information is available.

► 1 or 2 servings of fish weekly (not necessarily any more or less). Tuna fish in a can with spring water is fine. Stay away from canned fish packed in oil (vegetable oil). Other types of fish—such as salmon, mackerel, herring, mahi mahi, sardines, and whitefish—are fine too. If you are a sushi lover you're in luck—it's good for you! More good news—fish is also a great source of vitamin D. Don't obsess about this—simply make an effort to eat fish that you enjoy one or two times a week. If you prefer to eat it more frequently, by all means do so.

► 20% or less of your total daily calories should come from fat (not necessarily any less or more). This is an easy objective if you like to eat fruits, vegetables, fish, and lean meats. Fat may promote prostate cancer growth. Soy products, such as soy burgers or soy hotdogs, are usually low-fat. Turkey burgers, vegetable burgers, and other low-fat meats or meat substitutes are also good alternatives.

▶ Eat a variety of fruits and vegetables and fiber daily. Try not to focus on one type of fruit or vegetable. Mix them up! Blueberries, raspberries, tomatoes, broccoli, cauliflower, kale, pineapple . . . the list goes on and on. Pick your favorites and alternate them from day to day or week to week. A variety will hold your interest and additionally provide you with a vast array of anticancer compounds. Legumes or beans are another healthy choice for your diet. Navy, lima, soy, green . . . variety, variety, variety!

▶ Drink several cups of green tea weekly. Green tea research is impressive. One cup a day is a good place to start.

2. Exercise, Exercise, Exercise

Individuals who are more active may reduce their risk of prostate cancer. Light exercise, 3 or 4 times a week, is sufficient. Walk for 30 minutes at a time, jog, hike, swim, go rowing, walk on a treadmill, play golf . . . make it a part of your life.

3. Supplements

▶ 200 micrograms of selenium daily (in the form of selenomethionine)

▶ 50 to 100 IU of vitamin E daily (synthetic or natural)

▶ one general multivitamin daily (with at least 400 IU of vitamin D, 400 micrograms of folic acid, and a variety of the B-vitamins (niacin, B6, B12)

4. Remain Mentally Healthy

I cannot stress this enough. Socialize, meditate, exercise, reduce stress, keep life in perspective, get a massage, go on vacation, volunteer in the community, pursue your hobbies, laugh . . . do whatever you can to remain mentally healthy and happy. It is no secret that chronic mental depression may increase your risk of certain diseases. Always avoid or treat depression!

5. Prescription Drugs

Talk to your doctor. However, there are several drugs currently being tested that show potential for reducing the risk of prostate cancer.

6. Always Be Realistic—Everything in Moderation

Be good to yourself. Do not become obsessive about anything you do.

▶ Alcohol in moderation

▶ Do not smoke

When setting goals, ask yourself if you can implement the changes into your lifestyle on a permanent basis. If not, reassess and make adjustments in order to make your goals a permanent part of your daily routine. For example, if you set a goal of exercising 30 minutes a day, seven days a week, ask yourself if you will be able to achieve this on a regular basis. Setting goals you cannot achieve may cause you to become discouraged and quit altogether.

Do you enjoy a thick, juicy steak once in a while? How about a hot dog? In moderation, these are acceptable, for most individuals. As mentioned previously, your mental attitude has a great deal to do with your overall health. If you are happy and content after a good steak, hot dog, hamburger, etc., then you should certainly partake once in a while!

7. Have an Annual Physical Exam and Keep a Copy of Your Medical Records.

One of the best ways of beating cancer—and other serious disease—is through early detection. A yearly physical will let you know how you are doing overall. Your cholesterol level, blood pressure, PSA, and weight can be easily checked in one yearly visit. It may be the single most important thing you do to save your life. Early detection is the key to treatment of disease.

Keep a record of your own annual medical results so that you can compare them from year to year. Take control of your health!

Appendix of Supplement Interactions

Appendix of Supplement Interactions

Included is a list of various supplements and their possible negative interactions with other drugs. Please refer to individual chapters, when appropriate, within *The ABC's of Nutrition and Supplements for Prostate Cancer* for more specific information.

Never use any supplement without first discussing it with your doctor!

Supplement	Negative Effect
borage	Do not use in combination with anticonvulsant drugs.
bromelain (from pineapple)	Increases risk of bleeding when taken with anticoagulants.
echinacea	May counteract immune-suppressant drugs; may be toxic to the liver when taken in combination with anabolic steroids, ketoconazole, and antiandrogen drugs.
evening primrose oil	Do not use in combination with anticonvulsant drugs.
feverfew (for migraine headaches)	NSAIDs may reduce the effectiveness of feverfew. Increased risk of bleeding when used in combination with anticoagulants.
garlic	May enhance anticoagulant and antiplatelet drugs.
ginger	May enhance anticoagulant drugs.
ginkgo biloba	May enhance anticoagulant and antiplatelet drugs.

ginseng

May increase side effects of various stimulants. May enhance anticoagulant drugs. May also affect glucose levels—should not be used by diabetics. May interfere with digoxin monitoring.

grapefruit juice

Can be dangerous when used in combination with blood pressure medication (calcium channel blockers).

high-fiber herbs

May bind to drugs in the intestines, thereby delaying absorption of any medications taken at the same time.

kava kava

May result in coma when used in combination with alprazolam.

kelp

Contains iodine—may interfere with thyroid therapies.

licorice

May enhance effect of potassium-depleting drugs. May also increase time for effectiveness of corticosteroid drugs. May lower testosterone levels.

saw palmetto

May inhibit the absorption of iron.

St. John's Wort

Many different interactions with prescription drugs. May also increase the side effects of photosensitizing drugs, alcohol, and melatonin. May inhibit the absorption of iron.

zinc

Do not take with immunosuppressants.

Please talk to your doctor, check a Physician's Desk Reference (PDR) on herbal supplements, and ask about the latest information on side effects. Remember— if a supplement does not claim any side effects, it is either worthless or not enough information on its side effects is currently available.

Medical References

INTRODUCTION

Nelson, N.J. 1996. Is chemoprevention overrated or underfunded? J. National Cancer Institute 88: 947-949.

Smigel, K. 1997. International group releases first set of global dietary recommendations. J. National Cancer Institute 89:1570-1571.

Jacobs, J.J. 1997. Unproven alternative methods of cancer treatment. In Cancer: Principles and Practice of Oncology (5th edition), Eds: V.T. Devita, S. Hellman, and S.A. Rosenberg, 2993-3001. Philadelphia, PA: Lippincott-Raven.

Lippman, S.M., J.J. Lee, and A.L. Sabichi. 1998. Cancer chemoprevention: Progress and promise. J. National Cancer Institute 90:1514-1528.

Singh D.K., and S.M. Lippman. 1998. Cancer chemoprevention-Part I: Retinoids and carotenoids and other classic antioxidants. Oncology 12:1643-1658.

Singh, D.K., and S.M. Lippman. 1998. Cancer chemoprevention- Part II: Hormones, nonclassic antioxidant natural agents, NSAIDS, and other agents. Oncology 12:1787-1805.

Garay, C.A., and P.F. Engstrom. 1999. Chemoprevention of colorectal cancer: Dietary and pharmacologic approaches. Oncology 13:89-98.

Pienta, K.J., and P.S. Esper. 1993. Risk factors for prostate cancer. Annals of Internal Medicine 118:793-803. Fair, W.R., N.E. Fleshner, and W. Heston. 1997. Cancer of the prostate: A nutritional disease? Urology 50:840-848.

Moyad M.A., and K.J. Pienta, eds. 1999. Nontraditional cancer treatments. Special Issue of Seminars in Urologic Oncology 17:63-119.

CHAPTER 1

Neugut, A.I., D.J. Rosenberg, H. Ahsan, et al. 1998. Association between coronary heart disease and cancers of the breast, prostate, and colon. Cancer Epidemiology, Biomarkers & Prevention 7:869-873.

Rodriguez, C., E.E. Calle, L.M. Tatham, et al. 1998. Family history of breast cancer as a predictor for fatal prostate cancer. Epidemiology 9:525-529.

Tsubono, Y., T. Takahashi, Y. Iwase, et al. 1997. Dietary differences with green tea intake among middle-aged Japanese men and women. Preventive Medicine 26:704-710.

Klatsky, A.L. 1999. Is it the drink or the drinker? Circumstantial evidence only raises a probability. American Journal of Clinical Nutrition 69:2-3.

Lichtenstein, A.H., and L. Van Horn. 1998. Very low fat diets. Circulation 98:935-939.

Danesh, J., and P. Appleby. 1999. Coronary heart disease and iron status: meta-analyses of prospective studies. Circulation 99:852-854.

American Cancer Society. 1999. Cancer Facts & Figures. American Cancer Society, Atlanta, GA.

Dallongeville, J., N. Marecaux, J.C. Fruchart, and P. Amouyel. 1998. Cigarette smoking is associated with unhealthy patterns of nutrient intake: A meta-analysis. J. Nutrition 128:1450-1457.

Brown, K.M., P.C. Morrice, and G.G. Duthie. 1997. Erythrocyte vitamin E and plasma ascorbate concentrations in relation to erythrocyte peroxidation in smokers and nonsmokers: Dose response to vitamin E supplementation. American Journal of Clinical Nutrition 65:496-502.

Kujala, U.M., J. Kaprio, S. Sarna, and M. Koskenvuo. 1998. Relationship of leisure-time physical activity and mortality: The Finnish Twin Cohort. JAMA 279:440-444.

CHAPTER 2

Weissman, G. 1991. Aspirin. Scientific American 264:84-90.

Vane, J.R., R.J. Flower, and R.M. Botting. 1990. History of aspirin and its mechanism of action. Stroke 21:IV12-IV23.

Taketo, M.M. 1998. Cyclooxygenase-2 inhibitors in tumorigenesis (part I). J. National Cancer Institute 90:1529-1536.

Taketo, M.M. 1998. Cyclooxygenase-2 inhibitors in tumorigenesis (part II). J. National Cancer Institute 90: 1609-1620.

He, J., P.K. Whelton, B. Vu, and M.J. Klag. 1998. Aspirin and risk of hemorrhagic stroke: A meta-analysis of randomized controlled trials. JAMA 280:1930-1935.

Norrish, A.E., R.T. Jackson, and C.U. McRae. 1998. Non-steroidal anti-inflammatory drugs and prostate cancer progression. International Journal of Cancer 77:511-515

Anderson, K.M., T. Seed, M. Vos, et al. 1998. 5-Lipoxygenase inhibitors reduce PC-3 cell proliferation and initiate nonnecrotic cell death. The Prostate 37:161-173

Horan, A.H. 1998. Advances in angiogenesis research: Relevance to urological oncology. Journal of Urology 160:134-135.

Hejna, M., M. Raderer, and C.C. Zielinski. 1999. Inhibition of metastases by anticoagulants. J. National Cancer Institute 91:22-36.

Sturmer, T., R.J. Glynn, I.M. Lee, et al. 1998. Aspirin use and colorectal cancer: Post-trial follow-up data from the Physicians' Health Study. Annals of Internal Medicine 128: 713-720.

CHAPTER 3

Hartman, T.J., D. Albanes, P. Pietinen, et al. 1998. The association between baseline vitamin E, selenium, and prostate cancer in the alpha-tocopherol, beta-carotene cancer prevention study. Cancer Epidemiology, Biomarkers & Prevention 7:335-340.

Heinonen, O.P., D. Albanes, J. Virtamo, et al. 1998. Prostate cancer and supplementation with alpha-tocopherol and beta-carotene: Incidence and mortality in a controlled trial. J. National Cancer Institute 90:440-446.

Olson, K.B., and K.J. Pienta. 1998. Vitamins A and E: Further clues for prostate cancer prevention. J. National Cancer Institute 90:414-415.

Key, T.J., P.B. Silcocks, G.K. Davey, et al. 1997. A case-control study of diet and prostate cancer. British Journal of Cancer 76:678-687.

Nomura, A.M., G.N. Stemmermann, J. Lee, and N.E. Craft. 1997. Serum micronutrients and prostate cancer in Japanese Americans in Hawaii. Cancer Epidemiology, Biomarkers & Prevention 6:487-491.

Daviglus, M.L., A.R. Dyer, V. Persky, et al. 1996. Dietary beta-carotene, vitamin C, and risk of prostate cancer: Results from the Western Electric Study. Epidemiology 7:472-477.

Hall, A.K. 1996. Liarozole amplifies retinoid-induced apoptosis in human prostate cancer cells. Anti-Cancer Drugs 7:312-320.

van Poppel, G., and R.A. Goldbohm. 1995. Epidemiologic evidence for beta-carotene and cancer prevention. American Journal of Clinical Nutrition 62:1393S-1402S.

Giovannucci, E., A. Ascherio, E.B. Rimm, et al. 1995. Intake of carotenoids and retinol in relation to risk of prostate cancer. J. National Cancer Institute 87:1767-1776.

Ohno, Y., O. Yoshida, K. Oishi, et al. 1998. Dietary beta-carotene and cancer of the prostate: A case-control study in Kyoto, Japan. Cancer Research 48:1331-1336.

CHAPTER 4

Giovannucci, E., M.J. Stampfer, G.A. Colditz, et al. 1998. Multivitamin use, folate, and colon cancer in women in the Nurses' Health Study. Annals of Internal Medicine 129:517-524.

Vucenik, I., T. Kalebic, K. Tantivejkul, et al. 1998. Novel anticancer function of inositol hexaphosphate: Inhibition of human rhabdomyosarcoma in vitro and in vivo. Anticancer Research 18:1377-1384.

Boros, L.G., J.L. Brandes, W-N. Lee, et al. 1998. Thiamine supplementation to cancer patients: A double edged sword. Anticancer Research 18:595-602.

Shamsuddin, A.M., and G.Y. Yang. 1995. Inositol hexaphosphate inhibits growth and induces differentiation of PC-3 human prostate cancer cells. Carcinogenesis 16:1975-1979.

Shamsuddin, A.M., G. Yang, and I. Vucenik. 1996. Novel anti-cancer functions of IP6: Growth inhibition and differentiation of human mammary cancer cell lines in vitro. Anticancer Research 16:3287-3292.

Glynn, S.A., D. Albanes, P. Pietinen, et al. 1996. Colorectal cancer and folate status: A nested case-control study among male smokers. Cancer Epidemiology, Biomarkers & Prevention 5:487-494.

Giovanucci, E., E.B. Rimm, A. Ascherio, et al. 1995. Alcohol, low-methionine-low folate diets, and risk of colon cancer in men. J. National Cancer Institute 87:265-273.

White, E., J.S. Shannon, and R.E. Patterson. 1997. Relationship between vitamin and calcium supplement use and colon cancer. Cancer Epidemiology, Biomarkers & Prevention 6:769-774

Key, T.J.A., P.B. Silcocks, G.K. Davey, et al. 1997. A case-control study of diet and prostate cancer. British Journal of Cancer 76:678-687.

Vlajinac, H.D., J.M. Marinkovic, M.D. Ilic, and Kocev. 1997. Diet and prostate cancer: A case-control study. European Journal of Cancer 33:101-107.

CHAPTER 5

Folkers, K. 1996. Relevance of the biosynthesis of coenzyme Q10 and of the four bases of DNA as a rationale for the molecular causes of cancer and therapy. Biochemical and Biophysical Research Communications 224:358-361.

Landbo, C., and T.P. Almdal. 1998. Interaction between warfarin and coenzyme Q10. Ugeskrift for Laeger 160:3226-3227.

Lockwood, K., S. Moesgaard, and K. Folkers. 1994. Partial and complete regression of breast cancer in patients in relation to dosage of coenzyme Q10. Biochemical and Biophysical Research Communications 199:1504-1508.

Lockwood, K., S. Moesgaard, T. Hanioka, and K. Folkers. 1994. Apparent partial remission of breast cancer in high risk patients supplemented with nutritional antioxidants, essential fatty acids and coenzyme Q10. Molecular Aspects of Medicine 15:S231-S240.

Prieme, H., S. Loft, K. Nyyssonen, et al. 1997. No effect of supplementation with vitamin E, ascorbic acid, or coenzyme Q10 on oxidative DNA damage estimated by 8-oxo-7,8-dihydro-2'-deoxyguanosine excretion in smokers. American Journal of Clinical Nutrition 65:503-507.

Judy, W.V., R.A. Willis, and K. Folkers. 1998. Regression of prostate cancer and plasma specific antigens (PSA) in patients on treatment with COQ10. Proc. First Conference of the International Coenzyme Q10 Association. Abstract #143.

Yamamoto, Y., S. Yamashita, A. Fujisawa, et al. 1998. Oxidative stress in patients with hepatitis, cirrhosis, and hepatoma evaluated by plasma antioxidants. Biochemical & Biophysical Research Communications 247:166-170.

Yamamoto, Y., and S. Yamashita. 1997. Plasma ratio of ubiquinol and ubiquinone as a marker of oxidative stress. Molecular Aspects of Medicine 18:S79-S84.

Folkers, K., A. Osterborg, M. Nylander, et al. 1997. Activities of vitamin Q10 in animal models and a serious deficiency in patients with cancer. Biochemical and Biophysical Research Communications 234:296-299.

Larsson, O., and B.M. Johansson. 1987. Mevalonic acid products as mediators of cell proliferation in simian virus 40-transformed 3T3 cells. Cancer Research 47:4825-4829.

CHAPTER 6

Jones, J.A., A. Nguyen, M. Straub, et al. 1997. Use of DHEA in a patient with advanced prostate cancer: A case report and review. Urology 50:784-788.

Brzezinski, A. 1997. Mechanisms of disease: Melatonin in humans. NEJM 336:186-195.

Lissoni, P., M. Cazzaniga, G. Tancini, et al. 1997. Reversal of clinical resistance to LHRH analogue in metastatic prostate cancer by the pineal hormone melatonin: Efficacy of LHRH analogue plus melatonin in patients progressing on LHRH analogue alone. European Urology 31:178-181.

Mawson, A.R. 1998. Breast cancer in female flight attendants. Lancet 352:626.

Taverna, G., A. Trinchieri, A. Mandressi, et al. 1997. Variation in nocturnal urinary excretion of melatonin in a group of patients older than 55 years suffering from urogenital tract disorders. Archivio Italiano di Urologia, Andrologia 69:293-297.

Bartsch, C., and H. Bartsch. 1997. Significance of melatonin in malignant diseases. Wiener Klinische

Wochenschrift 109:722-729.

Philo, R., and A.S. Berkowitz. 1988. Inhibition of Dunning tumor growth by melatonin. Journal of Urology 139:1099-1102.

Buzzell, G.R. 1988. Studies on the effects of the pineal hormone melatonin on an androgen-insensitive rat prostatic adenocarcinoma, the Dunning R 3327 HIF tumor. J. Neural Transmission 72:131-140.

Neri, B., V. De Leonardis, M.T. Gemelli, et al. 1998. Melatonin as biological response modifier in cancer patients. Anticancer Research 18:1329-1332.

McNeil, C. 1997. Potential drug DHEA hits snags on way to clinic. J. National Cancer Institute 89:681-683.

CHAPTER 7

Kolonel, L.N., AM-Y. Nomura, and R.V. Cooney. 1999. Dietary fat and prostate cancer: Current status. J. National Cancer Institute 91:414-428.

Giovannucci, E., A. Ascherio, E.B. Rimm, et al. 1993. A prospective study of dietary fat and risk of prostate cancer. J. National Cancer Institute 85:1571-1579.

Kolonel, L.N., C.N. Yoshizawa, and J.H. Hankin. 1988. Diet and prostatic cancer: A case-control study in Hawaii. American Journal of Epidemiology 127:999-1012.

Zock, P.L., and M.B. Katan. 1998. Linoleic acid intake and cancer risk: A review and meta-analysis. American Journal of Clinical Nutrition 68:142-153.

Rose, D.P., and J.M. Connolly. 1991. Effects of fatty acids and eicosanoid synthesis inhibitors on the growth of two human prostate cancer cell lines. The Prostate 18:243-254.

Karmali, R.A., P. Reichel, L.A. Cohen, et al. 1987. The effects of dietary w-3 fatty acids on DU-145 transplantable human prostatic tumor. Anticancer Research 7:1173-1180.

Rose, D.P., and L.A. Cohen. 1988. Effects of dietary menhaden oil and retinyl acetate on the growth of DU-145 human prostatic adenocarcinoma cells transplanted into athymic nude mice. Carcinogenesis 9:603-605.

Mettlin, C., S. Selenskas, N. Natarajan, et al. 1989. Beta-carotene and animal fats and their relationship to prostate cancer risk. Cancer 64:605-612.

Pienta, K.J., H. Naik, A. Akhtar, et al. 1995. Inhibition of spontaneous metastasis in a rat prostate cancer model by oral administration of modified citrus pectin. J. National Cancer Institute 87:348-353.

Mills, P.K., W.L. Beeson, R.L. Phillips, et al. 1989. Cohort study of diet, lifestyle, and prostate cancer in Adventist men. Cancer 64:598-604.

CHAPTER 8

Tham, D.M., C.D. Gardner, and W.L. Haskell. 1998. Clinical Review 97-Potential health benefits of dietary phytoestrogens: A review of the clinical, epidemiological, and mechanistic evidence. J. of Endocrinology and Metabolism 83:2223-2235.

Nagata, C., N. Takatsuka, S. Inaba, et al. 1998. Effect of soymilk consumption on serum estrogen concentrations in premenopausal Japanese women. J. National Cancer Institute 90:1830-1835.

Herbert, JR., T.G. Hurley, B.C. Olendzki, et al. 1998. Nutritional and socioeconomic factors in relation to prostate cancer mortality: A cross-national study. J. National Cancer Institute 90:1637-1647.

Quak, S.H., and S.P. Tan. 1998. Use of soy-protein formulas and soyfood for feeding infants and children in Asia. American Journal of Clinical Nutrition 68:1444S-1446S.

Yan, L., J.A. Yee, D. Li, et al. 1998. Dietary flaxseed supplementation and experimental metastasis of melanoma cells in mice. Cancer Letters 124:181-186.

Orcheson, L.J., S.E. Rickard, M.M. Seidl, and L.U. Thompson. 1998. Flaxseed and its mammalian lignan precursor cause a lengthening or cessation of estrous cycling in rats. Cancer Letters 125:69-76.

Sung, M-K., M. Lautens, and L.U. Thompson. 1998. Mammalian lignans inhibit the growth of estrogen–independent human colon tumor cells. Anticancer Research 18:1405-1408.

Cunnane, S.C., M.J. Hamadeh, A.C. Liede, et al. 1995. Nutritional attributes of traditional flaxseed in healthy young adults. American Journal of Clinical Nutrition 61:62-68.

Wanasundara, P.K., and F. Shahidi. 1998. Process-induced compositional changes of flaxseed. Advances in Experimental Medicine & Biology 434:307-325.

Prasad, K., S.V. Mantha, A.D. Muir, and N.D. Westcott. 1998. Reduction of hypercholesterolemic atherosclerosis by CDC-flaxseed with very low alpha-linolenic acid. Atherosclerosis 136:367-375.

CHAPTER 9

Pinto, J.T., C. Qiao, J. Xing, et al. 1997. Effects of garlic thioallyl derivatives on growth, glutathione concentration, and polyamine formation of human prostate carcinoma cells in culture. American Journal of Clinical Nutrition 66:398-405.

Heber, D. 1997. The stinking rose: Organosulfur compounds and cancer. American Journal of Clinical Nutrition 66:425-426.

Dorant, E., P.A. van den Brandt, and R.A. Goldbohm. 1996. A prospective cohort study on the relationship between onion and leek consumption, garlic supplement use and the risk of colorectal carcinoma in The Netherlands. Carcinogenesis 17:477-484.

Dorant, E., P.A. van den Brandt, and R.A. Goldbohm. 1994. A prospective cohort study on Allium vegetable consumption, garlic supplement use, and the risk of lung carcinoma in The Netherlands. Cancer Research 54:6148-6153.

Dorant, E., P.A. van den Brandt, and R.A. Goldbohm. 1995. Allium vegetable consumption, garlic supplement intake, and female breast carcinoma incidence. Breast Cancer Research & Treatment 33:163-170.

Sigounas, G., J. Hooker, A. Anagnostou, and M. Steiner. 1997. S-allylmercaptocysteine inhibits cell proliferation and reduces the viability of erythroleukemia, breast, and prostate cancer cell lines. Nutrition & Cancer 27:186-191.

Key, T.J., P.B. Silcocks, G.K. Davey, et al. 1997. A case-control study of diet and prostate cancer. British Journal of Cancer 76:678-687.

Dorant, E., P.A. van den Brandt, R.A. Goldbohm, et al. 1993. Garlic and its significance for the prevention of cancer in humans: A critical view. British Journal of Cancer 67:424-429.

Simons, L.A., S. Balasubramaniam, M. von Konigsmark, et al. 1995. On the effect of garlic on plasma lipids and lipoproteins in mild hypercholesterolaemia. Atherosclerosis 113:219-225.

Isaacsohn, J.L., M. Moser, E.A. Stein, et al. 1998. Garlic powder and plasma lipids and lipoproteins. Archives of Internal Medicine 158:1189-1194.

CHAPTER 10

Giovannucci, E. 1999. Tomatoes, tomato-based products, lycopene, and cancer: Review of the epidemiologic literature. J. National Cancer Institute 91:317-331.

Clinton, S.K. 1998. Lycopene: Chemistry, biology, and implications for human health and disease. Nutrition Reviews 56:35-51.

Mills, P.K., L. Beeson, R.L. Phillips, and G.E. Fraser. 1989. Cohort study of diet, lifestyle, and prostate cancer in Adventist men. Cancer 64:598-604.

Franceschi, S., E. Bidoli, C. La Vecchia, et al. 1994. Tomatoes and risk of digestive-tract cancers. International Journal of Cancer 59:181-184.

Giovannucci, E., A. Ascherio, E.B. Rimm, et al. 1995. Intake of carotenoids and retinol in relation to risk of prostate cancer. J. National Cancer Institute 87:1767-1776.

Levy, J., E. Bosin, B. Feldman, et al. 1995. Lycopene is a more potent inhibitor of human cancer cell proliferation than either alpha-carotene or beta-carotene. Nutrition & Cancer 24:257-266.

Stahl, W., and H. Sies. 1992. Uptake of lycopene and its geometrical isomers is greater from heat-processed than from unprocessed tomato juice in humans. Journal of Nutrition 122:2161-2166.

Di Mascio, P., S. Kaiser, and H. Sies. 1989. Lycopene as the most efficient biological carotenoid singlet oxygen quencher. Archives of Biochemistry and Biophysics 274:532-538.

Rentzepis, M.J., H. Newmark, M. Lipkin, et al. 1998. Lycopene does not inhibit the growth of subcutaneously implanted LNCaP tumor cells in nude mice: Implications for chemoprevention. Journal of Urology

159:13 (abstract 49).

Pastori, M., H. Pfander, D. Boscoboinik, and A. Azzi. 1998. Lycopene in association with alpha-tocopherol inhibits at physiological concentrations proliferation of prostate carcinoma cells. Biochemical and Biophysical Research Communications 250:582-585.

CHAPTER 11

Hsieh, T.C., S.S. Chen, X. Wang, et al. 1997. Regulation of androgen receptor (AR) and prostatic specific antigen (PSA) expression in the androgen-responsive human prostate LNCaP cells by ethanolic extracts of the Chinese herbal preparation PC-SPES. Biochemical & Molecular Biology International 42:535-544.

Halicka, H.D., B. Ardelt, G. Juan, et al. 1997. Apoptosis and cell cycle effects induced by extracts of the Chinese herbal preparation PC-SPES. International Journal of Oncology 11:437-448.

Zava, D.T., C.M. Dollbaum, and M. Blen. 1998. Estrogen and progestin bioactivity of foods, herbs, and spices. Proc. Society for Experimental Biology & Medicine 217:369-378.

DiPaola, R.S., H. Zhang, G.H. Lambert, et al. 1998. Clinical and biologic activity of an estrogenic herbal combination (PC-SPES) in prostate cancer. NEJM 339:785-791.

The Leuprolide Study Group. 1984. Leuprolide versus diethylstilbestrol for metastatic prostate cancer. NEJM 311:1281-1286.

Bishop, M.C. 1996. Experience with low-dose oestrogen in the treatment of advanced prostate cancer: A personal view. British Journal of Urology 78:921-928.

Sigurjonsdottir, H.A., J. Ragnarsson, L. Franzson, et al. 1995. Is blood pressure commonly raised by moderate consumption of licorice? J. Human Hypertension 9:345-348.

Rossner, S., P-O. Hedlund, T. Joestrand, et al. 1985. Treatment of prostatic cancer: effects on serum lipoproteins and the cardiovascular system. Journal of Urology 133:53-57.

Aprikian, A.G., W.R. Fair, V.E. Reuter, et al. 1994. Experience with neoadjuvant diethylstilbestrol and radical prostatectomy in patients with locally advanced prostate cancer. British Journal of Urology 74:630-636.

Moyad, M.A., K.J. Pienta, and J.E. Montie. 1999. Use of PC-SPES, a commercially available supplement for prostate cancer, in a patient with hormone-naive disease. Urology 54:319-323.

CHAPTER 12

Clement, P. 1998. Lessons from basic research in selenium and cancer prevention. J. Nutrition 128:1845-1854.

Gonzalez, J.A., K.M. Kernen, K.M. Peters, et al. 1998. The oral administration of powdered shark cartilage for the treatment of advanced prostate cancer. Michigan Urological Association Annual Meeting Presentation.

Coppes, M.J., R.A. Anderson, M.R. Egeler, and J.E.A. Wolff. 1998. Alternative therapies for the treatment of childhood cancer. NEJM 339:846-847.

Simone, C.B., N.L. Simone, and C.B. II Simone. 1998. Shark cartilage for cancer. Lancet 351:1440.

Dupont, E., P.E. Savard, C. Jourdain, et al. 1998. Antiangiogenic properties of a novel shark cartilage extract: potential role in the treatment of psoriasis. J. Cutaneous Medicine and Surgery 2:146-152.

Fontenele, J.B., G.S. Viana, J. Xavier-Filho, and J.W. de-Alencar. 1996. Anti-inflammatory and analgesic activity of a water-soluble fraction from shark cartilage. Brazilian Journal of Medical & Biological Research 29:643-646.

Nelson, M.A., B.W. Porterfield, E.T. Jacobs, and L.C. Clark. 1999. Selenium and prostate cancer prevention. Seminars in Urologic Oncology 17:91-96.

Clark, L.C., G.F. Combs, B.W. Turnbull, et al. 1996. Effects of selenium supplementation for cancer prevention in patients with carcinoma of the skin. JAMA 276:1957-1963.

Colditz, G.A. 1996. Selenium and cancer prevention. JAMA 276:1984-1985.

Yoshizawa, K., W.C. Willet, S.J. Morris, et al. 1998. Study of prediagnostic selenium level in toenails and the risk of advanced prostate cancer. J. National Cancer Institute 90:1219-1224.

Fairweather-Tait, S.J. 1997. Bioavailability of selenium. European Journal of Clinical Nutrition 51:S20-S23.

Fleet, J.C., and J. Mayer. 1997. Dietary selenium repletion may reduce cancer incidence in people at high risk who live in areas with low soil selenium. Nutrition Reviews 55:277-279.

Redman, C., J.A. Scott, A.T. Baines, et al. 1998. Inhibitory effect of selenomethionine on the growth of three selected human tumor cell lines. Cancer Letters 125:103-110.

Russo, M.W., S.C. Murray, J.I. Wurzelmann, et al. 1997. Plasma selenium levels and the risk of colorectal adenomas. Nutrition and Cancer 28:125-129.

Garland, M., S. Morris, M.J. Stampfer, et al. 1995. Prospective study of toenail selenium levels and cancer among women. J. National Cancer Institute 87:497-505.

CHAPTER 13

Miller, D.R., G.T. Anderson, J.J. Stark, et al. 1998. Phase I/II trial of the safety and efficacy of shark cartilage in the treatment of advanced cancer. J. Clinical Oncology 16:3649-3655.

Brem, H., and J. Folkman. 1975. Inhibition of tumor angiogenesis mediated by cartilage. J. Experimental Medicine 141:427-439.

Lee, A., and R. Langer. 1983. Shark cartilage contains inhibitors of tumor angiogenesis. Science 221:1185-1187. 60 minutes/CBS television. 1993. Segment 2/28/93 Broadcast: Shark Cartilage.

Asher, B., and E. Vargo. 1996. Possible link between shark cartilage and hepatitis. Annals of Internal Medicine 125:780-781.

Gonzalez, J.A., K.M. Kernen, K.M. Peters, et al. 1998. The oral administration of powdered shark cartilage for the treatment of advanced prostate cancer. Michigan Urological Association Annual Meeting Presentation.

Coppes, M.J., R.A. Anderson, M.R. Egeler, and J.E.A. Wolff. 1998. Alternative therapies for the treatment of childhood cancer. NEJM 339:846-847.

Simone, C.B., N.L. Simone, and C.B. II Simone. 1998. Shark cartilage for cancer. Lancet 351:1440.

Dupont, E., P.E. Savard, C. Jourdain, et al. 1998. Antiangiogenic properties of a novel shark cartilage extract: potential role in the treatment of psoriasis. J. Cutaneous Medicine and Surgery 2:146-152.

Fontenele, J.B., G.S. Viana, J. Xavier-Filho, and J.W. de-Alencar. 1996. Anti-inflammatory and analgesic activity of a water-soluble fraction from shark cartilage. Brazilian Journal of Medical & Biological Research 29:643-646.

CHAPTER 14

NCI, DCPC Chemoprevention Branch and Agent Development Committee. 1996. Clinical development plan: Tea extracts green tea polyphenols epigallocatechin gallate. J. Cellular Biochemistry 26S:236-257.

Chung, F-I.., M. Wnag, A. Rivenson, et al. 1998. Inhibition of lung carcinogenesis by black tea in Fischer rats treated with a tobacco-specific carcinogen: Caffeine as an important constituent. Cancer Research 58:4096-4101.

Jankun, J., S.H. Selman, and R. Swiercz. 1997. Why drinking green tea could prevent cancer. Nature 387:561.

Heilbrun, L.K., A. Nomura, and G.N. Stemmermann. 1986. Black tea consumption and cancer risk: A prospective study. British Journal of Cancer 54:677-683.

Ahmad, N., D.K. Feyes, A-L. Nieminen, et al. 1997. Green tea constituent epigallocatechin-3-gallate and induction of apoptosis and cell cycle arrest in human carcinoma cells. J. National Cancer Institute 89:1881-1886.

Matsumoto, N., T. Kohri, K. Okushio, and Y. Hara. 1996. Inhibitory effects of tea catechins, black tea extract and oolong tea extract on hepatocarcinogenesis. Japanese Journal of Cancer Research 87:1034-1038.

Kaegi, E. 1998. Unconventional therapies for cancer: 1. Essiac. Canadian Medical Association Journal 158:897-902.

Kohlmeier, L., K.G.-C. Weterings, S. Steck, and F.J. Kok. 1997. Tea and cancer prevention: An evaluation of the epidemiologic literature. Nutrition and Cancer 27:1-13.

Nakachi, K., K. Suemasu, K. Suga, et al. 1998. Influence of drinking green tea on breast cancer malignancy among Japanese patients. Japanese Journal of Cancer Research 89:254-261.

Sadzuka, Y., T. Sugiyama, and S. Hirota. 1998. Modulation of cancer chemotherapy by green tea. Clinical Cancer Research 4:153-156.

CHAPTER 15

Moertel, C.G., T.R. Fleming, E.T. Creagan, et al. 1985. High-dose vitamin C versus placebo in the treatment of patients with advanced cancer who have had no prior chemotherapy: A randomized double-blind comparison. NEJM 312:137-141.

Creagan, E.T., C.G. Moertel, J.R. O'Fallon, et al. 1979. Failure of high-dose vitamin C (ascorbic acid) therapy to benefit patients with advanced cancer. A controlled trial. NEJM 301:687-690.

Maramag, C., M. Menon, K.C. Balaji, et al. 1997. Effect of vitamin C on prostate cancer cells in vitro: Effect on cell number, viability, and DNA synthesis. The Prostate 32:188-195.

Venugopal, M., J.M. Jamison, J. Gilloteaux, et al. 1996. Synergistic antitumor activity of vitamins C and K3 against human prostate carcinoma cell lines. Cell Biology International 20:787-797.

Shane, B. 1997. Vitamin C pharmacokinetics: It's dÈj‡ vu all over again. American Journal of Clinical Nutrition 66:1061-1062.

Blanchard, J., T.N. Tozer, and M. Rowland. 1997. Pharmacokinetic perspectives on megadoses of ascorbic acid. American Journal of Clinical Nutrition 66:1165-1171.

Podmore, I.D., H.R. Griffiths, K.E. Herbert, et al. 1998. Vitamin C exhibits pro-oxidant properties. Nature 392:559-561.

Jacques, P.F., A. Taylor, S.E. Hankinson, et al. 1997. Long-term vitamin C supplement use and prevalence of early age-related lens opacities. American Journal of Clinical Nutrition 66:911-916.

Cameron, E. 1991. Protocol for the use of vitamin C in the treatment of cancer. Medical Hypothesis 36:190-194.

Jacob, R.A. 1998. Vitamin C nutriture and risk of atherosclerotic heart disease. Nutrition Reviews 56:334-340.

CHAPTER 16

van den Berg, H. 1997. Bioavailability of vitamin D. European Journal of Clinical Nutrition 51:S76-S79.

Thomas, M.K., D.M. Lloyd-Jones, R.I. Thadhani, et al. 1998. Hypovitaminosis D in medical patients. NEJM 338:777-783.

Konety, B.R., C.S. Johnson, D.L. Trump, and R.H. Getzenberg. 1999. Vitamin D in the prevention and treatment of prostate cancer. Seminars in Urologic Oncology 17:77-84.

Dawson-Hughes, B., G.E. Dallal, E.A. Krall, et al. 1991. Effect of vitamin D supplementation on wintertime and overall bone loss in healthy postmenopausal women. Annals of Internal Medicine 115:505-512.

Light, B.W., W.D. Yu, Z.R. Shurin, et al. 1998. Potentiation of paclitaxel-mediated anti-tumor activity with 1,25-dihydoxycholecalciferol (1,25-D3). Proc. AACR 39:308 (abstract 2105).

Getzenberg, R.H., B.W. Light, P.R. Lapco, et al. 1997. Vitamin D inhibition of prostate adenocarcinoma growth and metastasis in the Dunning rat prostate model system. Urology 50:999-1006.

Schwartz, G.G., T.A. Oeler, M.R. Uskokovic, and R.R. Bahnson. 1994. Human prostate cancer cells: Inhibition of proliferation by vitamin D analogs. Anticancer Research 14:1077-1082.

Chen, T.C., Q. Shao, H. Heath III, and M.F. Holick. 1993. An update on the vitamin D content of fortified milk from the United States and Canada. NEJM 329:1507.

Hanchette, C.L., and G.G. Scwartz. 1992. Geographic patterns of prostate cancer mortality: Evidence for a protective effect of ultraviolet radiation. Cancer 70:2861-2869.

Giovannucci, E., E.B. Rimm, A. Wolk, et al. 1998. Calcium and fructose intake in relation to risk of prostate cancer. Cancer Research 58:442-447.

CHAPTER 17

Moyad, M.A., S.K. Brumfield, and K.J. Pienta. 1999. Vitamin E, alpha- and gamma- tocopherol and prostate cancer. Seminars in Urologic Oncology 17:85-90.

Wolf, G. 1998. Gamma-tocopherol: an efficient protector of lipids against nitric oxide-initiated peroxidative damage. Nutrition Reviews 55:376-378.

Tran, K., and A.C. Chan. 1992. Comparative uptake of alpha- and gamma-tocopherol by human endothelial cells. Lipids 27:38-41.

Christen, S., A.A. Woodall, M.K. Shigenaga, et al. 1997. Gamma-tocopherol traps mutagenic electrophiles such as NOx and complements alpha-tocopherol: Physiological implications. PNAS 94:3217-3222.

Sigounas, G., A. Anagnostou, and M. Steiner. 1997. dl-alpha-Tocopherol induces apoptosis in erythroleukemia, prostate, and breast cancer cells. Nutrition and Cancer 28:30-35.

Kushi, L.H., A.R. Folsom, R.J. Prineas, et al. 1996. Dietary antioxidant vitamins and death from coronary heart disease in postmenopausal women. NEJM 334:1156-1162.

Gann, P.H., J. Ma, E. Giovannucci, et al. 1999. Lower prostate cancer risk in men with elevated plasma lycopene levels: Results of a prospective analysis. Cancer Research 59:1225-1230.

Cohn, W. 1997. Bioavailability of vitamin E. European Journal of Clinical Nutrition 51:S80-S85.

Stone, W.L., and A.M. Papas. 1997. Tocopherols and the etiology of colon cancer. J. National Cancer Institute 89:1006-1014.

Heinonen, O.P., D. Albanes, J. Virtamo, et al. 1998. Prostate cancer and supplementation with alpha-tocopherol and beta-carotene: Incidence and mortality in a controlled trial. J. National Cancer Institute 90:440-446.

CHAPTER 18

Costello, L.C., and R.B. Franklin. 1998. Novel role of zinc in the regulation of prostate citrate metabolism and its implications in prostate cancer. The Prostate 35:285-296.

Iguchi, K., M. Hamatake, R. Ishida, et al. 1998. Induction of necrosis by zinc in prostate carcinoma cells and identification of proteins increased in association with this induction. European Journal of Biochemistry 253:766-770.

Lekili, M., A. Ergen, and I. Celebi. 1991. Zinc plasma levels in prostatic carcinoma and BPH. International Urology and Nephrology 23:151-154.

Macknin, M.L., M. Piedmonte, C. Calendine, et al. 1998. Zinc gluconate lozenges for treating the common cold in children: A randomized controlled trial. JAMA 279:1962-1967.

Ogunlewe, J.O., and D.N. Osegbe. 1989. Zinc and cadmium concentrations in indigenous blacks with normal, hypertrophic, and malignant prostate. Cancer 63:1388-1392.

Chandra, R.K. 1984. Excessive intake of zinc impairs immune responses. JAMA 252:1443-1146.

Anonymous. 1980. Zinc and immunocompetence. Nutrition Reviews 38:288-289.

Leake, A., G.D. Chrisholm, A. Busuttil, and F.K. Habib. 1984. Subcellular distribution of zinc in the benign and malignant human prostate: Evidence for a direct zinc androgen interaction. Acta Endocrinologica 105:281-288.

Sandstrom, B. 1997. Bioavailability of zinc. European Journal of Clinical Nutrition 51:S17-S19.

Key, T.J., P.B. Silcocks, G.K. Davey, et al. 1997. A case-control study of diet and prostate cancer. British Journal of Cancer 76: 678-687.

CHAPTER 19

Eisenberg, D.M., R.B. Davis, S.L. Ettner, et al. 1998. Trends in alternative medicine use in the United States, 1990-1997: Results of a follow-up national survey. JAMA 280:1569-1575.

Morey, S.S. 1998. NIH issues consensus statement on acupuncture. American Family Physician 57:2545-2546.

Li, Q.S., S.H. Cao, G.M. Xie, et al. 1994. Combined traditional Chinese medicine and Western medicine. Relieving effects of Chinese herbs, ear-acupuncture, and epidural morphine on postoperative pain in liver cancer. Chinese Medical Journal 107:289-294.

Honjo, H., H. Kitakoji, K. Kawakita, et al. 1998. Acupuncture for urinary incontinence in patients with chronic spinal cord injury. Japanese Journal of Urology 89:665-669.

Yamashita, H., H. Tsukayama, Y. Tanno, et al. 1998. Adverse effects related to acupuncture. JAMA 280:1563-1564.

Wong, A.H-C., M. Smith, and H.S. Boon. 1998. Herbal remedies in psychiatric practice. Archives of

General Psychiatry 55:1033-1044.

Sikora, R., M.H. Sohn, F-J. Deutz, et al. 1989. Ginkgo biloba extract in the therapy of erectile dysfunction. Journal of Urology 141:188A (abstract 73).

Sikora, R., M.H. Sohn, B. Engelke, et al. 1998. Randomized placebo-controlled study on the effects of oral treatment with Ginkgo biloba extract in patients with erectile dysfunction. Journal of Urology 159:240A (abstract 917).

Hammar, M., J. Frisk, O. Grimas, et al. 1998. Acupuncture treatment of vasomotor symptoms in men with prostatic carcinoma: A pilot study. Journal of Urology 161:853-856.

Bone, K. 1993/1994. Kava: A safe herbal treatment for anxiety. British Journal of Phytotherapy 3:147-153.

CHAPTER 20

Katiyar, S.K., N.J. Korman, H. Mukhtar, and R. Agarwal. 1997. Protective effects of Silymarin against photocarcinogenesis in a mouse skin model. J. National Cancer Institute 89:556-566.

Relman, A.S. 1982. Closing the books on Laetrile. NEJM. 306:236.

Kaegi, E. 1998. Unconventional therapies for cancer: 714-X. Canadian Medical Association Journal 158:1621-1624.

Kaegi, E. 1998. Unconventional therapies for cancer: Iscador. Canadian Medical Association Journal 158:1157-1159.

Kaegi, E. 1998. Unconventional therapies for cancer: Hydrazine sulfate. Canadian Medical Association Journal 158:1327-1330.

Bustamante, J., J.K. Lodge, L. Marcocci, et al. 1998. Alpha-lipoic acid in liver metabolism and disease. Free Radical Biology & Medicine 24:1023-1039.

Giovannucci, E., M. Leitzman, D. Spiegelman, et al. 1998. A prospective study of physical activity and prostate cancer in male health professionals. Cancer Research 58:5117-5122.

Heber, D., I. Yip, J.M. Ashley, et al. 1999. Cholesterol-lowering effects of a proprietary Chinese red-yeast-rice dietary supplement. American J. Clinical Nutrition 69:231-236.

Garzon, P., and M.J. Eisenberg. 1998. Variation in the mineral content of commercially available bottled waters: Implications for health and disease. The American J. Medicine 105:125-130.

Croyle, R.T. 1998. Depression as a risk factor for cancer: Renewing a debate on the psychobiology of disease. J. National Cancer Institute 90:1856-1857.

CHAPTER 21

Stephens, F.O. 1997. Phytoestrogens and prostate cancer: Possible preventive role. Medical Journal of Australia 167:138-140.

Kreinhoff, U., I. Elmadfa, F. Salomon, and B. Weidler. 1990. Antioxidant status after surgical stress. Infusionstherapie (Basel) 17:261-267.

Ornish, D.M., P. Carroll, E.B. Pettengill, et al. 1998. Can lifestyle changes reverse prostate cancer? Journal of Urology 159:218 (abstract 842).

Carter, J.P., G.P. Sace, V. Newbode, et al. 1993. Dietary management may improve survival from nutritionally linked cancers based on analysis of representative cases. J. American College of Nutrition 12:209-226.

Ashley, J., W. Aronson, I. Yip, et al. 1997. Acceptance of a low fat, high fiber diet with soy protein supplement in men with prostate cancer. Proc. 16th International Congress of Nutrition 271 PT 533.

Yip, I., W. Aronson, R. Elashoff, et al. 1998-1999. Nutrition adjuvant therapy for treatment of prostate cancer. Experimental Biology, In press.

Yip, I., D. Heber, and W. Aronson. 1999. Nutrition and prostate cancer. Urologic Clinics of North America 26:403-411.

Nakachi, K., K. Suga, Y. Higashi, and K. Imai. 1998. Influence of drinking green tea on breast cancer malignancy among Japanese patients. Proc. AACR 39:89 (abstract 604).

Massion, A.O., J. Teas, J.R. Hebert, et al. 1995. Meditation, melatonin and breast/prostate cancer: Hypothesis and preliminary data. Medical Hypothesis 44:39-46.

Ai, A.L., C. Peterson, and S.F. Bolling. 1997. Psychological recovery from coronary artery bypass graft surgery: The use of complementary therapies. J. Alternative & Complementary Medicine 3:343-353.

CHAPTER 22

Wilt, T.J., A. Ishani, G. Stark, et al. 1998. Saw palmetto extracts for treatment of benign prostatic hyperplasia. JAMA 280:1604-1609.

Dutkiewicz, S. 1996. Usefulness of Cernilton in the treatment of benign prostatic hyperplasia. J. International Urology & Nephrology 28:49-53.

Rugendorff, E.W., W. Weidner, L. Ebeling, and A.C. Buck. 1993. Results of treatment with pollen extract (Cernilton N) in chronic prostatitis and prostatodynia. British Journal of Urology 71:433-438.

Suzuki T, K. Kurokawa, T. Mashimo, et al. 1992. Clinical effect of Cernilton in chronic prostatitis. Hinyokika Kiyo-Acta Urologica Japonica 38:489-494.

Buck, A.C., R. Cox, R.W. Rees, et al. 1990. Treatment of outflow tract obstruction due to benign prostatic hyperplasia with the pollen extract, Cernilton. A double-blind, placebo-controlled study. British Journal of Urology 66:398-404.

Maekawa, M., T. Kishimoto, R. Yasumoto, et al. 1990. Clinical evaluation of Cernilton on benign prostatic hypertrophy-A multiple center double-blind study with Paraprost. Hinyokika Kiyo-Acta Urologica Japonica 36:495-516.

Di Silverio, F., S. Monti, A. Sciarra, et al. 1998. Effects of long-term treatment with Serenoa repens (Permixon) on the concentrations and regional distribution of androgens and epidermal growth factor in benign prostatic hyperplasia. The Prostate 37:77-83.

Lowe, F.C., K. Dreikorn, A. Borkowski, et al. 1998. Review of placebo-controlled trials utilizing phytotherapeutic agents for treatment of BPH. The Prostate 37:187-193.

Dreikorn, K., A. Borkowski, J. Braeckman, et al. 1998. Other medical therapies. In Proceedings of the Fourth International Consultation on BPH; July 2-5, 1997, Eds. L. Denis, K. Griffiths, S. Khoury, et al., 633-659. Plymouth, UK: Health Publications, Ltd.

Marks, L.S., and V.E. Tyler. 1999. Saw palmetto extract: newest (and oldest) treatment alternative for men with symptomatic benign prostatic hyperplasia. Urology 53:457-461.

Glossary & Index

abdomen
the part of the body below the ribs and above the pelvic bone, which contains the intestines, liver, kidneys, stomach, bladder, and prostate

ablation
reduction of—for example, in the management of prostate cancer

adenocarcinoma
a form of cancer that develops from a malignant abnormality in the cells lining a glandular organ such as the prostate; almost all prostate cancers are adenocarcinomas

adjuvant
an additional treatment used to increase the effectiveness of the primary therapy; radiation therapy and hormonal therapy are often used as adjuvant treatments following a radical prostatectomy

adrenal glands
the two adrenal glands are located above the kidneys; they produce a variety of different hormones, including sex hormones—the adrenal androgens

adrenalectomy
the surgical removal of one or both adrenal glands

age-adjusted
modified to take account of the age of an individual or group of individuals; for example, prostate cancer survival data and average normal PSA values can be adjusted according to the ages of groups of men

alkaline phosphatase
an enzyme in blood, bone, kidney, spleen, and lungs; used to detect bone or liver metastasis

alpha-blockers
pharmaceuticals that act on the prostate by relaxing certain types of muscle tissue; these pharmaceuticals are often used in the treatment of BPH

analog
a synthetic chemical or pharmaceutical that behaves very like a normal chemical in the body, e.g., LHRH analogs

Anandron
trade or brand name for nilutamide

Androcur
trade name for cyproterone, an antiandrogen

androgen
a hormone that is responsible for male characteristics and the development and function of male sexual organs (e.g., testosterone) produced mainly by the testicles but also in the cortex of the adrenal glands

anesthetic
a drug that produces general or local loss of physical sensations, particularly pain; a "spinal" is the injection of a local anesthetic into the area surrounding the spinal cord

aneuploid
having an abnormal number of sets of chromosomes; for example, tetraploid means having two paired sets of chromosomes, which is twice as many as normal; aneuploid cancer cells tend not to respond well to hormone therapy; See also diploid

angiogenesis
the formation of new blood vessels; a characteristic of tumors

anterior
the front; for example, the anterior of the prostate faces forward

antiandrogen
a compound (usually a synthetic pharmaceutical) that blocks or otherwise interferes with the normal action of androgens at cellular receptor sites

antiandrogen withdrawal response (AAWR)
a decrease in PSA caused by the withdrawal of an antiandrogen such as Casodex or flutamide after CHT begins to fail; occurs when there are PCa cells that have mutated to feed on the antiandrogen rather than T and DHT; withdrawal kills those cells

antibiotic
a pharmaceutical that can kill certain types of bacteria

antibody
protein produced by the immune system as a defense

against an invading or "foreign" material or substance (an antigen); for example, when you get a cold, your body produces antibodies to the cold virus

anticoagulant
a pharmaceutical that helps stop blood from clotting

antigen
"foreign" material introduced into the body (a virus or bacterium, for example) or other material that the immune system considers to be "foreign" because it is not part of the body's normal biology (e.g., prostate cancer cells)

anus
the opening of the rectum

apex
the tip or bottom of the prostate, e.g., the part of the prostate farthest away from the bladder

aspiration
the use of suction to remove fluid or tissue, usually through a fine needle (e.g., aspiration biopsy)

asymptomatic
having no recognizable symptoms of a particular disorder

autologous
one's own; for example, autologous blood is a patient's own blood which is removed prior to surgery in case a patient needs a transfusion during or after surgery

base
the base of the prostate is the wide part at the top of the prostate closest to the bladder

benign
relatively harmless; not cancerous; not malignant

benign prostate hyperplasia (BPH)
a noncancerous condition of the prostate that results in the growth of both glandular and stromal (supporting connective) tumorous tissue, enlarging the prostate and obstructing urination; See prostatitis

benign prostatic hypertrophy (BPH)
similar to benign prostatic hyperplasia, but caused by an increase in the size of cells rather than the growth of more cells

bicalutamide
a nonsteroidal antiandrogen available in the United States and some European countries for the treatment of prostate cancer; also known as Casodex

bilateral
both sides; for example, a bilateral orchidectomy is a procedure in which both testicles are removed, and a bilateral adrenalectomy is an operation in which both adrenal glands are removed

biopsy
sampling of tissue from a particular part of the body (e.g., the prostate) in order to check for abnormalities such as cancer; in the case of prostate cancer, biopsies are usually carried out under ultrasound guidance using a specially designed device known as a prostate biopsy gun; removed tissue is typically examined microscopically by a pathologist in order to make a precise diagnosis of the patient's condition

bladder
the hollow organ in which urine is collected and stored in the body

blood chemistry
measured concentrations of many chemicals in the blood; abnormal values can indicate spread of cancer or side effects of therapy

blood count
analysis of blood cells and platelets; abnormal values can indicate cancer in the bone or side effects of therapy

bone marrow
soft tissue in bone cavities that produces blood cells

bone scan
a technique more sensitive than conventional X-rays that uses a radiolabeled agent to identify abnormal or cancerous growths within or attached to bone; in the case of prostate cancer, a bone scan is used to identify bony metastases, which are definitive for cancer that has escaped from the prostate; metastases appear as "hot spots" on the film; however,

the absence of "hot spots" does not prove the absence of tiny metastases

bowel preparation
the cleaning of the bowels or intestines, which is normal prior to abdominal surgery such as radical prostatectomy

BPH
See benign prostate hyperplasia — benign prostatic hypertrophy

brachytherapy
a form of radiation therapy in which radioactive seeds or pellets that emit radiation are implanted in order to kill surrounding tissue (e.g., the prostate, including prostate cancer cells)

CAB, complete androgen blockade
See CHT

cancer
the growth of abnormal cells in the body in an uncontrolled manner; unlike benign tumors, these tend to invade surrounding tissues and spread to distant sites of the body via the bloodstream and lymphatic system

capsule
the fibrous tissue that acts as an outer lining of the prostate

carcinoma
a form of cancer that originates in tissues that line or cover a particular organ; See adenocarcinoma

Casodex
brand or trade name of bicalutamide

castration
the use of surgical or medical techniques to eliminate testosterone produced by the testes

CAT scan, Computerized Axial Tomography (also CT)
a method of combing images from multiple X-rays under the control of a computer to produce cross-sectional or three-dimensional pictures of the internal organs that can be used to identify abnormalities; the CAT scan can identify prostate enlarge-ment, but is not always effective for assessing the stage of prostate cancer; for evaluating metastases of the lymph nodes or more distant soft tissue sites, the CAT scan is significantly more accurate

catheter
a hollow (usually flexible plastic) tube that can be used to drain fluids from or inject fluids into the body; in the case of prostate cancer, it is common for patients to have a transurethral catheter to drain urine for some time after treatment by surgery or some forms of radiation therapy

CDUS
color-flow Doppler ultrasound; an ultrasound method that more clearly images tumors by observing the Doppler shift in sound waves caused by the rapid flow of blood through tiny blood vessels that are characteristic of tumors

CGA, Chromogtanin A
a small cell prostate cancer or neuroendocrine cell marker

CHB, combination hormone blockade:
same as CHT or ADT (androgen deprivation therapy or MAB (maximal androgen blockade) usually involving an LHRH agonist and an antiandrogen

chemotherapy
the use of pharmaceuticals or other chemicals to kill cancer cells; in many cases chemotherapeutic agents kill not only cancer cells but also other cells in the body, which makes such agents potentially very dangerous

CHT, combined hormonal therapy
the use of more than one hormone in therapy; especially the use of LHRH analogs (e.g., Lupron, Zoladex) to block the production of testosterone by the testes, plus antiandrogens, e.g., Casodex (bicalutamide), Eulexin (flutamide), Anadron (nilutamide), or Androcur (cyproterone) to compete with DHT and T (testosterone) for cell sites, thereby depriving cancer cells of DHT and T needed for growth

clinical trial
a carefully planned experiment to evaluate a treatment or a medication (often a new pharmaceutical) for an unproven use; Phase I trials are very prelimi-

nary short-term trials involving a few patients to see if drugs have any activity or any serious side effects; Phase II trials may involve 20 to 50 patients and are designed to estimate the most active dose of a new drug and determine its side effects; Phase III trials involve many patients and compare a new therapy against the current standard or best available therapy

complication therapy
See CHT or CHB

complication
an unexpected or unwanted effect of a treatment, pharmaceutical, or other procedure

conformational therapy
the use of careful planning and delivery techniques designed to focus radiation on the areas of the prostate and surrounding tissue that need treatment and to protect areas that do not need treatment; three-dimensional conformational therapy is a more sophisticated form of this method

contracture
scarring that can occur at the bladder neck after a radical prostatectomy and that results in narrowing of the passage between the bladder and the urethra

corpora cavernosa
the part of a man's penis that fills with blood when he is sexually excited, giving the organ the stiffness required for intercourse

corpora spongiosum
a spongy chamber in a man's penis that fills with blood when he is sexually excited, giving the organ the stiffness required for intercourse

cryoablation
See cryosurgery

cryosurgery
the use of liquid nitrogen probes to freeze a particular organ to extremely low temperatures to kill the tissue, including any cancerous tissue; when used to treat prostate cancer, the cryoprobes are guided by transrectal ultrasound

cryotherapy
See cryosurgery

CT Scan, computerized or computed tomography
See CAT scan

cyproterone
an antiandrogen

cystoscope
an instrument used by physicians to look inside the bladder and the urethra

cystoscopy
the use of a cystoscope to look inside the bladder and the urethra

cytokines
growth factors important to cellular function

debulking
reduction of the volume of cancer by one of several techniques; most frequently used to imply surgical debulking

DES
See diethylstilbestrol

DHT
See dihydrotestosterone

diagnosis
the evaluation of signs, symptoms, and selected test results by a physician to determine the physical and biological causes of the signs and symptoms and whether a specific disease or disorder is involved

diethylstilbestrol
a female hormone commonly used for treatment of prostate cancer

digital rectal examination
the use by a physican of a lubricated and gloved finger inserted into the rectum to feel for abnormalities of the prostate and rectum

dihydrotestosterone (DHT) (5 alpha dihydrotestosterone)
the male hormone that is most active in the prostate; it is manufactured when an enzyme (5 alpha reductase) in the prostate stimulates the transformation of testosterone to DHT

differentiation
the use of the differences between prostate cancer cells when seen under the microscope as a method to grade the severity of the disease; well-differentiated cells are easily recognized as normal cells, while poorly differentiated cells are abnormal, cancerous, and difficult to recognize as belonging to any particular type of cell group

diploid
having one complete set of normally paired chromosomes, i.e., a normal amount of DNA; diploid cancer cells tend to grow slowly and respond well to hormone therapy

DNA
deoxyribonucleic acid; the basic biologically active chemical that defines the physical development and growth of nearly all living organisms

double-blind
a form of clinical trial in which neither the physician nor the patient knows the actual treatment any individual patient is receiving; double-blind trials are a way of minimizing the effects of the personal opinions of patients and physicians on the results of the trial

doubling time
the time that it takes a particular focus of cancer to double in size

downsizing
the use of hormonal or other forms of management to reduce the volume of prostate cancer in and/or around the prostate prior to attempted curative treatment

downstaging
the use of hormonal or other forms of management in the attempt to lower the clinical stage of

prostate cancer prior to attempted curative treatment (e.g., from stage T3a to stage T2b); this technique is highly controversial

DRE
See digital rectal examination

dysplasia
See PIN

dysuria
urination that is problematic or painful

edema
swelling or accumulation of fluid in some part of the body

ejaculatory ducts
the tubular passages through which semen reaches the prostatic urethra during orgasm

erectile dysfunction
See impotence

Emcyt
the brand or trade name of estramustine phosphate in the United States

endogenous
naturally inherent to the organism

estramustine phosphate
a chemotherapeutic agent used in the treatment of some patients with late-stage prostate cancer

estrogen
a female hormone; certain estrogens (e.g., diethylstilbestrol) are used by some physicans for treatment of prostate cancer

Eulexin
the brand or trade name of flutamide in the United States

experimental
an unproven (or even untested) technique or procedure; note that certain experimental treatments are commonly used in the management of prostate cancer

267

external radiation therapy (also external beam therapy)
a form of radiation therapy in which the radiation is delivered by a machine pointed at the area to be radiated

false negative
an erroneous negative test result; for example, an imaging test that fails to show the presence of a cancer tumor later found by biopsy is said to have returned a false negative result

false positive
a positive test result mistakenly identifying a state or condition that does not in fact exist

finasteride
an inhibitor of the enzyme (5 alpha reductase) that stimulates the conversion of testosterone to DHT; used to treat BPH

flare reaction
A temporary increase in tumor growth and symptoms caused by LHRH agonists; can be mild to dangerous; may be prevented by taking an antiandrogen (Casodex) several days before starting LHRH agonist (Lupron or Zoladex)

flow cytometry
a measurement method that determines the fraction of cells that are diploid, tetraploid, aneuploid, etc.

flutamide
an antiandrogen used in the palliative hormonal treatment of advanced prostate cancer and sometimes in the adjuvant and neoadjuvant hormonal treatment of earlier stages of prostate cancer; normal dosage is two capsules every eight hours (not just at meals)

frequency
the need to urinate often

frozen section
a technique in which removed tissue is frozen, cut into thin slices, and stained for microscopic examination; a pathologist can rapidly complete a frozen section analysis; for this reason it is commonly used during surgery to quickly provide the surgeon with vital information, such as a preliminary patho-

logic opinion of the presence or absence of prostate cancer (usually in the pelvic lymph nodes)

gastrointestinal
related to the digestive system and/or the intestines

genital system
the biological system which (in males) includes the testicles, vas deferens, prostate, and penis

genitourinary system
the combined genital and urinary systems; also known as the genitourinary tract

gland
a structure or organ that produces a substance used in another part of the body

Gleason
name of physician who developed the Gleason grading system commonly used to grade prostate cancer

Gleason score
a widely used method for classifying the cellular differentiation of cancerous tissues; the less the cancerous cells appear like normal cells, the more malignant the cancer; two numbers, each from 1 to 5, are assigned successively to the two most predominant patterns of differentiation present in the examined tissue sample and are added together to produce the Gleason score; high numbers indicate poor differentiation and therefore cancer

GNRH, genadotropin-releasing hormone
See LHRH analogs

goserelin acetate
a luteinizing hormone-releasing hormone analog used In the palliative hormonal treatment of advanced prostate cancer and sometimes in the adjuvant and neoadjuvant hormonal treatment of earlier stages of prostate cancer

grade
a means of describing the potential degree of severity of a cancer based on the appearance of cancer cells under a microscope; See Gleason score

gynecomastia
enlargement or tenderness of the male breasts or

nipples—a possible side effect of hormonal therapy

hematospermia
the occurrence of blood in the semen

hematuria
the occurance of blood in the urine

heredity
the historical distribution of biological characteristics in a group of related individuals via their DNA

hereditary
inherited from one's parents and earlier generations

histology
the study of the appearance and behavior of tissue, usually carried out under a microscope by a pathologist (who is a physician) or a histologist (who is not necessarily a physician)

hormones
biologically active chemicals that are responsible for the development of secondary sexual characteristics

hormone therapy
the use of hormones, hormone analogs, and certain surgical techniques to treat disease (in this case advanced prostate cancer) either on their own or in combination with other hormones or in combination with other methods of treatment; because prostate cancer is usually dependent on male hormones to grow, hormonal therapy can be an effective means of alleviating symptoms and retarding the development of the disease

hot flash
the sudden sensation of warmth in the face, neck, and upper body—a side effect of many forms of hormone therapy

hypercalcemia
abnormally high concentrations of calcium in the blood

hyperplasia
enlargement of an organ or tissue because of an increase in the number of cells in that organ or tissue; See also BPH

hyperthermia
treatment that uses heat—for example, heat produced by microwave radiation

imaging
a technique or method allowing a physician to see something that would not normally be visible

immune system
the biological system that protects a person or animal from the effects of foreign materials, such as bacteria, cancer cells, and other things that might make that person or animal sick

implant
a device that is inserted into the body—e.g., a tiny container of radioactive material inserted in or near a tumor; also, a device inserted in order to replace or substitute for an ability that has been lost; for example, a penile implant is a device that can be surgically inserted into the penis to provide rigidity for intercourse

impotence
the inability to have or to maintain an erection

incidental
insignificant or irrelevant; for example, incidental prostate cancer (also known as latent prostate cancer) is a form of prostate cancer that is of no clinical significance to the patient in whom it is discovered

incontinence (urinary)
loss of urinary control; there are various kinds and degrees of incontinence; overflow incontinence is a condition in which the bladder retains urine after voiding; as a consequence, the bladder remains full most of the time, resulting in involuntary seepage of urine from the bladder; stress incontinence is the involuntary discharge of urine when there is increased pressure upon the bladder, as in coughing or straining to lift heavy objects; total incontinence is the inability to voluntarily excerise control over the sphincters of the bladder neck and urethra, resulting in total loss of retentive ability

indication
a reason for doing something or taking some action; also used to mean the approved clinical application of a pharmaceutical

inflammation
any form of swelling, pain, or irritation

informed consent
permission to proceed given by a patient after being fully informed of the purposes and potential consequences of a medical procedure

interferon
a body protein that affects antibody production and that can modulate (regulate) the immune system

interstitial
within a particular organ; for example, interstitial prostate radiation therapy is radiation therapy applied within the prostate using implanted radioactive pellets or seeds; See also brachytherapy

intravenous
into a vein

invasive
requiring an incision or the insertion of an instrument or substance into the body

investigational
a drug or procedure allowed by the FDA for use in clinical trials

IVP (intravenous pyelogram)
a procedure that introduces an X-ray-absorbing dye into the urinary tract in order to allow the physician to view a superior image of the tract by taking an X-ray; used to check for the spread of cancer to the kidneys and bladder

Kegel exercises:
a set of exercises designed to improve the strength of the muscles used in urinating

kidney
one of a pair of organs whose primary function is to filter the fluids passing through the body

laparoscopy
a technique that allows the physician to observe internal organs through an optical device inserted directly into the body through a small surgical incision

latent
insignificant or irrelevant; for example, latent prostate cancer (also known as incidental prostate cancer) is a form of prostate cancer that is of no clinical significance to the patient

leuprolide acetate
an LHRH analog

LHRH
See luteinizing hormone-releasing hormone

LHRH analogs (or agonists)
synthetic compounds that are chemically similar to luteinizing hormone-releasing hormone (LHRH), but are sufficiently different that they suppress testicular production of testosterone by binding to the LHRH receptor in the pituitary gland; they either have no biological activity and therefore competitively inhibit the action of LHRH, or they have LHRH activity that exhausts the production of LH by the pituitary; used in the palliative hormonal treatment of advanced prostate cancer and sometimes in the adjuvant and neoadjuvant hormonal treatment of earlier stages of prostate cancer

libido
interest in sexual activity

LNCap:
a line of human prostate cancer cells used in laboratory studies; this cell line is hormonally dependent

lobe
one of the two sides of an organ that clearly has two sides (e.g., the prostate or the brain)

localized
restricted to a well-defined area

lupron
the United States trade or brand name of Leuprolide Acetate, an LHRH agonist

luteinizing hormone-releasing hormone (LHRH)
a hormone responsible for stimulating the production of testosterone in the body

lymph (also lymphatic) fluid
the clear fluid in which all of the cells in the body are

constantly bathed; carries cells that help fight infection

lymph nodes
the small glands that occur throughout the body that filter the clear fluid known as lymph or lymphatic fluid; lymph nodes filter out bacteria and other toxins, as well as cancer cells

lymphadenectomy
also known as a pelvic lymph node dissection, this procedure involves the removal and microscopic examination of selected lymph nodes, a common site of metastatic disease with prostate cancer; this procedure can be performed during surgery prior to the removal of the prostate gland, or by means of a small incision a "laparoscopic lymphadenectomy" may be performed—a simple operation requiring only an overnight stay in the hospital

lymphatic system
the tissue and organs that produce, store, and carry cells that fight infection; includes bone marrow, spleen, thymus, lymph nodes, and channels that carry lymph fluid

MAB (maximal androgen blockade)
See CHT, CHB

MAD (maximal androgen deprivation)
See CHB,CHT

magnetic resonance
absorption of specific frequencies of radio and microwave radiation by atoms placed in a strong magnetic field

magnetic resonance imaging (MRI)
the use of magnetic resonance with atoms in body tissues to produce distinct cross-sectional, and even three-dimensional images of internal organs; MRI is primarily of use in staging biopsy-proven prostate cancer

malignancy
a growth or tumor composed of cancerous cells

malignant
cancerous; tending to become progressively worse and to result in death; having the invasive and metastatic (spreading) properties of cancer

margin
normally used to mean the "surgical margin," which is the outer edge of the tissue removed during surgery; if the surgical margin shows no sign of cancer ("negative margins"), then the prognosis is good

medical oncologist
an oncologist primarily trained in the use of medicines (rather than surgery) to treat cancer

metastasize
to spread to other parts of the body

metastatic
having the characteristics of a secondary tumor

metastatic workup
a group of tests, including bone scans, X-rays, and blood tests, to ascertain whether cancer has metastasized

Metastron
the brand or trade name of Strontium-89 in the United States

misstaging
the assignment of an incorrect clinical stage at initial diagnosis because of the difficulty of assessing the available information with accuracy

monoclonal
formed from a single group of identical cells

MRI
See magnetic resonance imaging

morbidity
unhealthy consequences and complications resulting from treatment

negative
the term used to describe a test result that does not show the presence of the substance or material for which the test was carried out; for example, a negative bone scan would show no sign of bone metastasis

neoadjuvant
added before; for example, neoadjuvant hormone therapy is hormone therapy given prior to another

271

form of treatment, such as a radical prostatectomy

neoplasia
the growth of cells under conditions that would tend to prevent the development of normal tissue (e.g., a cancer)

nerve sparing
term used to describe a type of prostatectomy in which the surgeon saves the nerves that affect sexual and related functions

nilutamide
an antiandrogen; still experimental in the United States, but available in Canada and some other countries

nocturia
the need to urinate frequently at night

noninvasive
not requiring any incision or the insertion of an instrument or substance into the body

NSE (neuron-specific enolase)
a neuroendocrine marker; See CGA

oncologist
a physician who specializes in the treatment of various types of cancer

oncology
the branch of medical science dealing with tumors; an oncologist is a specialist in the study of cancerous tumors

orchiectomy
the surgical removal of one or both testicles

organ
a group of tissues that work in concert to carry out a specific set of functions (e.g., the heart, lungs, or prostate)

osteoblast
a cell that forms bone

osteoclast
a cell that breaks down bone cells, grows in bone tissue, and apparently absorbs bone tissue

osteolysis
destruction of bone

overstaging
the assignment of an overly high clinical stage at initial diagnosis because of the difficulty of assessing the available information with accuracy (e.g., Stage T3b as opposed to Stage T2b)

palliative
designed to relieve a particular problem without necessarily solving it; for example, palliative therapy is given in order to relieve symptoms and improve quality of life, but does not cure the patient

palpable
capable of being felt during a physical examination by an experienced physician; in the case of prostate cancer, this normally refers to some form of abnormality of the prostate that can be felt during a digital rectal examination

PAP (prostatic acid phosphatase)
an enzyme now measured only rarely to decide whether prostate cancer has escaped from the prostate

pathologist
a physician who specializes in the examination of tissues and blood samples to help decide which diseases are present and how they should be treated

PDQ (physician's data query)
an NCI-supported database available to physicians, containing current information on standard treatments and ongoing clinical trials

pelvis
that part of the skeleton that joins the lower limbs of the body together

penile
of the penis

penis
the male organ used in urination and intercourse

perineal
of the perineum

perineum
the area of the body between the scrotum and the rectum; a perineal procedure utilizes this area as the point of entry

perioheral
outside the central region

PET scan
Positron emission tomography using a radioactive isotope that is taken up by tumor tissue showing that the tumor is functional; current studies do not indicate a high utility of PET scanning in prostate cancer that is newly diagnosed, perhaps related to the usual slow doubling times

PIN (prostatic intraepithelial [or intraductal] neoplasia)
a pathologically identifiable condition believed to be a possible precursor of prostate cancer, also known by many physicians as dysplasia

placebo
a form of safe but nonactive treatment frequently used as a basis for comparison with pharmaceuticals in research studies

ploidy
a term used to describe the number of sets of chromosomes in a cell; See also diploid and aneuploid

positive
the term used to describe a test result that shows the presence of the substance or material for which the test was carried out; for example, a positive bone scan would show signs of bone metastasis

posterior
toward the rear; for example, the posterior of the prostate faces a man's back

prognosis
the patient's potential clinical outlook based on the status and probable course of his disease; chance of recovery

progression
continuing growth or regrowth of the cancer

prolactin (PRL)
a trophic hormone produced by the pituitary that increases androgen receptors, increases sensitivity to androgens, and regulates production and secretion of citrate

Proscar
brand name of finasteride

prostascint
a monoclonal antibody test directed against the Prostate Specific Membrane Antigen (PSMA); seems to focus on androgen-independent tumor tissue

prostate
the gland surrounding the urethra and immediately below the bladder in males

prostatectomy
surgical removal of part or all of the prostate gland

prostate-specific antigen
See PSA

prostatic acid phosphatase
See PAP

prostatitis
infection or inflammation of the prostate gland, treatable by medication and/or manipulation; (BPH is a more permanent laying down of fibroblasts and connective tissue caused when the prostate tries to contain a relatively silent chronic lower-grade infection, often requiring a TURP to relieve the symptoms)

prosthesis
a man-made device used to replace a normal body part or function

protocol
a precise set of methods by which a research study is to be carried out

PSA (Prostate-Specific Antigen)
a protein secreted by the epithelial cells of the prostate gland, including cancer cells; an elevated level in the blood indicates an abnormal condition of the prostate gland, either benign or malignant; it is used to detect potential problems in the prostate gland and to follow the progress of PCA Therapy; See screening

PSA-II
(Prostate-Specific Antigen Type II Assay), reports the percentage of free-PSA to total-PSA (total PSA = free PSA + bound PSA); helpful for screening purposes when PSA values are above the normal threshold for an age group and less than 10; one study showed that men with PSA II > 25% had no PCa; those with <10% were likely to have PCa; not yet FDA approved (as of 4/96), but available

PSA RT-PCR (PSA Reverse Transcriptase Polymerase Chain Reaction)
a blood test that detects micrometastatic cells circulating in the bloodstream; may be useful as a screening tool to help avoid unnecessary invasive treatments (RP, RT, etc.,) for patients with metastasized PCa; not FDA approved

PSM (Prostate-Specific Membrane)
a membrane that surrounds the protoplasm (cytoplasm) of prostate cells

PSMA
prostate-specific membrane antigen

quality of life
an evaluation of health status relative to the patient's age, expectations, and physical and mental capabilities

radiation oncologist
a physician who has received special training regarding the treatment of cancers with different types of radiation

radiation therapy (RT)
the use of X-rays and other forms of radiation to destroy malignant cells and tissue

radical
(in a surgical sense) directed at the cause of a disease; thus radical prostatectomy is the surgical removal of the prostate with the intent to cure the problem believed to be caused by or within the prostate

radical prostatectomy
an operation to remove the entire prostate gland and seminal vesicles

radioisotope
a type of atom (or a chemical that is made up of a type of atom) that emits radioactivity

radiosensitivity
the degree to which a type of cancer responds to radiation therapy

radiotherapy
See radiation therapy

randomized
the process of assigning patients in a random manner to different forms of treatment in a research study

rectal exam
See digital rectal exam

rectum
the final part of the intestines, which ends at the anus

recurrence
the reappearance of disease

refractory
resistant to therapy; e.g., hormone refractory prostate cancer is resistant to forms of treatment based on the use of hormones

regression
reduction in the size of a single tumor or reduction in the number and/or size of several tumors

remission
the real or apparent disappearance of some or all of the signs and symptoms of cancer; the period (temporary or permanent) during which a disease remains under control, without progressing; even complete remission does not necessarily indicate cure

resection
surgical removal

resectoscope
instrument inserted through the urethra used by a urologist to remove tissue (usually from the prostate) that allows the physician to actually see precisely where he or she is cutting

resistance:
(in a medical sense) a patient's ability to fight off a

disease as a result of the effectiveness of the patient's immune system

response
a decrease in disease that occurs because of treatment

retention
difficulty in initiation of urination or the inability to completely empty the bladder

retropublic prostatectomy
surgical removal of the prostate through an incision in the abdomen

risk
the chance or probability that a particular event will or will not happen

RP
See radical prostatectomy

RTCPR
See RT-PCR

RT-PCR (reverse transcriptase polymerase chain reaction)
a technique that allows a physician to search for tiny quantities of protein, such as PSA, in the blood or other fluids and tissues; See PSA

salvage
a procedure intended to "rescue" a patient following the failure of a prior treatment; for example, a salvage prostatectomy would be the surgical removal of the prostate after the failure of prior radiation therapy or cryosurgery

scrotum
the pouch of skin containing the testicles

screening
separating patients with tumors from those without tumors; multiple criteria are often used; the following PSA screening "cutoff" levels for PCa are replacing the older 4.0 value:

Age	PSA "Cutoff" (ng/mL)
40-49	up to 2.5
50-59	up to 3.5
60-69	up to 4.5
70-79	up to 6.5

secondary to
derived from or consequent to a primary event or thing

selenium
a relatively rare nonmetallic element found in food in small quantities that may have some role in prevention of cancer

semen
the whitish, opaque fluid emitted by a male at ejaculation

seminal
related to the semen; for example, the seminal vesicles are glands at the base of the bladder and connected to the prostate that provide nutrients for the semen

sensitivity
the probability that a diagnostic test can correctly identify the presence of a particular disease, assuming the test was properly conducted; specifically, the number of true positive results divided by the sum of the true positive results and the false negative results; See specificity

sextant
having six parts; thus, a sextant biopsy is a biopsy that takes six samples

side effect
a reaction to a medication or treatment (most commonly used to mean an unnecessary or undesirable effect)

sign
physical changes that can be observed as a consequence of an illness or disease

specificity
the probability that a diagnostic test can correctly identify the absence of a particular disease, assuming the test was properly conducted; specifically, the number of true negative results divided by the sum of the true negative results and the false positive results; a method that detects 95% of true PCa cases is highly sensitive, but if it also falsely indicates that 40% of those who do not have PCa do

have PCa then its specificity is 60%—rather poor

stage

a term used to define the size and physical extent of a cancer

staging

the process of assigning a stage in a specific patient in light of all the available information; it is used to help determine appropriate therapy; there are two staging methods: the Whitmore-Jewett staging classification (1956) and the more detailed TNM (Tumor, Nodes, Metastases) classification (1992) of the American Joint Committee on Cancer and the International Union Against Cancer; staging should be subcategorized as clinical staging and pathologic staging; pathologic stage usually relates to what is found at the time of surgery; Stage A is a clinically undetectable tumor confined to the gland and is an incidental finding at prostate surgery

Stage A (Whitmore-Jewett) becomes T1 (TNM)
Stage B becomes T2
Stage C becomes T3

Whitmore-Jewett stages

Stage A is a clinically undetectable tumor confined to the gland and is an incidental finding at prostate surgery

A1: well-differentiated with focal involvement
A2: moderately or poorly differentiated or involves multiple foci in the gland

Stage B is a tumor confined to the prostate gland

B0: nonpalpable, PSA-detected
B1: single nodule in one lobe of the prostate
B2: more extensive involvement of one lobe or involvement of both lobes

Stage C is a tumor clinically localized to the periprostatic area but extending through the prostatic capsule; seminal vesicles may be involved.

C1: clinical extracapsular extension
C2: extracapsular tumor producing bladder outlet or ureteral obstruction
Stage D is metastatic disease
D0: clinically localized disease (prostate only) but persistently elevated enzymatic serum acid phosphatase
D1: regional lymph nodes only
D2: distant lymph nodes, metastases to bone or visceral organs
D3: D2 prostate cancer patients who relapse after adequate endocrine therapy

TNM Stages

Primary Tumor (T)
TX: Primary tumor cannot be assessed
T0: No evidence of primary tumor
T1: Clinically nonapparent tumor not palpable or visible by imaging
T1a: Tumor incidental histologic finding in 5% or less of tissue resected
T1b: Tumor incidental histologic finding in more 5 % of tissue resected
T1c: Tumor identified by needle biopsy (e.g., because of elevated PSA)
T2: Tumor confined within the prostate
T2a: Tumor involves half of a lobe or less
T2b: Tumor involves more than half a lobe, but not both lobes
T2c: Tumor involves both lobes
T3: Tumor extends through the prostatic capsule
T3a: Unilateral extracapsular extension
T3b: Bilateral extracapsular extension
T3c: Tumor invades the seminal vesicle(s)
T4: Tumor is fixed or invades adjacent structures other than the seminal vesicles
T4a: Tumor invades any of bladder neck, external sphincter, or rectum
T4b: Tumor invades levator muscles and/or is fixed to the pelvic wall

Regional Lymph Nodes (N)

NX: Regional lymph nodes cannot be assessed
N0: No regional lymph node metastasis
N1: Metastasis in a single lymph node, 2 cm or less in greatest dimension
N2: Metastasis in a single lymph node, more than 2 cm but not more than 5 cm in greatest dimension; or multiple lymph node metastases, none more than 5 cm in greatest dimension
N3: Metastases in a lymph node more than 5 cm in greatest dimension
Distant Metastases (M)

MX: Presence of distant metastasis cannot be assessed
M0: No distant metastasis
M1: Distant metastasis
M1a: Nonregional lymph node(s)
M1b: Bone(s)
M1c: Other site(s)

stent
a tube used by a surgeon to drain fluids

stricture
scarring as a result of a procedure or an injury that constricts the flow of urine through the urethra

strontium-89
an injectable radioactive product used to relieve bone pain for some patients with prostate cancer that no longer responds to hormones or appropriate forms of chemotherapy

subcapsular
under the capsule; for example, a subcapsular orchiectomy is a form of castration in which the contents of each testicle are removed but the testicular capsules are then closed and remain in the scrotum

suture
surgical stitching used in the closure of a cut or incision

symptom
a feeling, sensation, or experience associated with or resulting from a physical or mental disorder and noticeable by the patient

systemic
throughout the whole body

testis
one of two male reproductive glands located inside the scrotum that are the primary sources of the male hormone testosterone

testicle
See testis
testosterone (T)
the male hormone or androgen which comprises most of the androgens in a man's body; chiefly pro-duced by the testicles; may be produced in tissues from precursors such as androstenedione; testosterone is essential to complete male sexual function and fertility

therapy
the treatment of disease or disability

TNM (tumor, nodes, metastases)
See staging

transition
change; for example, the transition zone of the prostate is the area of the prostate closest to the urethra and has features that distinguish it from the much larger peripheral zone

transperineal
through the perineum

transrectal
through the rectum

transurethral
through the urethra

treatment
administration of remedies to a patient for a disease

TRUS (transrectal ultrasound)
a method that uses echoes of ultrasound waves (far beyond the hearing range) to image the prostate by inserting an ultrasound probe into the rectum; commonly used to visualize prostate biopsy procedures

TRUS-P
See TRUS

tumor
an excessive growth of cells caused by uncontrolled and disorderly cell replacement; an abnormal tissue growth that can be either benign or malignant; See benign; malignant)

TURP (transurethral resection of the prostate)
a surgical procedure to remove tissue obstructing the urethra; the technique involves the insertion of an instrument called a resectoscope into the penile urethra, and is intended to relieve obstruction of urine flow due to enlargement of the prostate

TUR/P
See TURP

ultrasound
sound waves at a particular frequency (far beyond the hearing range) whose echoes bouncing off tissue can be used to image internal organs (or a baby in the womb)

understaging
the assignment of an overly low clinical stage at initial diagnosis because of the difficulty of assessing the available information with accuracy (e.g., Stage T2b as opposed to Stage T3b)

unit
a surgical term for a pint (usually of blood)

ureter
an anatomical tube that drains urine from one of the two kidneys to the bladder

urethra
the tube that drains urine from the bladder through the prostate and out through the penis

urgency
the need to urinate very soon

urinary system
the group of organs and their interconnections that permits excess, filtered fluids to exit the body, including (in the male) the kidneys, the ureters, the bladder, the urethra, and the penis

urologist
a doctor trained first as a surgeon who specializes in disorders of the genitourinary system

UTI (urinary tract infection)
an infection identifiable by the presence of bacteria (or theoretically viruses) in the urine; may be associated with a fever or a burning sensation on urination

vas deferens
tube through which sperm travel from the testes to the prostate prior to ejaculation

vasectomy
operation to make a man sterile by cutting the vas

deferens, thus preventing passage of sperm from the testes to the prostate

vesicle
a small sac containing a biologically important fluid

watchful waiting
active observation and regular monitoring of a patient without actual treatment

Whitmore-Jewett staging
See staging

X-ray
a type of high-energy radiation that can be used at low levels to make images of the internal structures of the body and at high levels for radiation therapy

Zoladex
trade or brand name for goserelin acetate, an LHRH agonist

zone
part or area of an organ